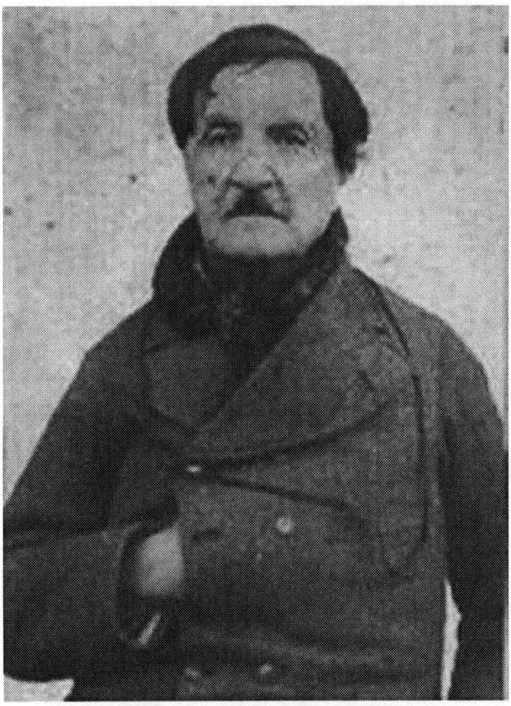

Count Cesare Mattei
(A Rare Photograph from the Collection of Editor)

Cesare Mattei
Electro-Homeopathy

Cesare Mattei's

Principles of Electro Homeopathy

Interpreted & Revised

By

Dr. Debasish Kundu

Originals

Delhi

First Published by:
Lake View Medical Institute and Sanitarium,
Depot for Electro-Homeopathic Remedies and Books
1619 Diversey Avenue, Chicago, Illinois, 1885

Revised Edition Published 2017

ISBN 13: 978-81-8454-197-7

ISBN 10: 81-8454-197-X

Published By
Originals
A-6, Second Floor, Nimri Commercial Centre,
Ashok Vihar Phase-4, Delhi - 110 052 (India)
Tel.: +91 11 2730 2453 Fax: 011 4706 1936
Website: www.Lppindia.com
e-mail: info@Lppindia.com

Printed At
D K Fine Art Press P Ltd.
Delhi-110052

Printed in India

Prof. Dr. Debasish Kundu

M.D.H., F.F.Hom, F.I.H.M.S., Ph.D.(U.S.A.), D.Sc. (Colombo)

Fellow of International Holistic Medical Society, CA, U.S.A.

Fellow of Foundation of Homeopathy, MO, U.S.A.

Fellow of World E.Homeopathy System of Medical Council, Hong Kong

Faculty, International Holistic Medical Society, CA, U.S.A.

Faculty, Association of Independent Natural Science Schools Colleges, Professions & Arts, MO, U.S.A.

Vice-President, American Nutritional Medical Association, CA, U.S.A.

Foreign Bureau Chief (India), Holistic Medical Hylite International, CA, U.S.A.

Visiting Professor, Khulna Homeopathic Medical College & Hospital, Khulna, Bangladesh

Ex-Director General, Mooreland University, U.S.A.

Former Adjunct. Faculty & Associate Professor, Department of Human Behavior, Newport University, U.S.A.

Editor In Chief, International Journal of Homeopathy & Natural Medicines, USA

Editor in Chief, The Internet Journal of Herbal and Plant Medicine, USA

Author,

Diseases of Women,

Natural Medicines,

A Clinical Treatise on Cancer,

Aids & Homeopathy,

Pharmacodynamics,

Aids & Your Sex Life,

Aids & Homeopathy,

Essentials of Acupuncture,

Materia Medica for the New Age Man, etc.

Recipient, Royal Assyrian Order of Merit (OIUCM, 1993)

Laureate, United Nations Dag Hammarskjold Award for Medicine (1995)

Recipient, Special Achievement Award, International Conference on E. Omeopatia, Poretta Terme, Bologna, Italy (2008)

Preface

There has been demand from the fraternity for an edition that is written in simple English, not so demanding of resource books for words and phrases and idioms of 18th century, since the English translations of Cesare Mattei's books have been done vastly by clergymen with rich English of that golden era, the translated versions often demand a good command of English besides encyclopedias and dictionaries.

It is an attempt to Rewrite the book in simple language with much needed Interpretation & Revision. The entire text has been thoroughly revised and rewritten, in some places the original French edition has been consulted, also enriched with footnotes wherever necessary.

Cover the true wisdom with 'fantastic veil'.

Dr. Debasish Kundu
drdkundu@msn.com
22 September, 2017

Contents

Electro-Homeopathy

An Introduction

General Idea of the New Science, its Importance, Progress, Struggles and Future of the New Discovery

Wisdom is the result of the knowledge

of things that were hidden.- Job*

During twenty years I have worked to spread my discovery; I have reason to believe that at my death it will be known to the whole world. I have the pleasure to acquaint all honest persons, interested in my existence, that my death, so often reported in many large cities, is not a fact. Neither am I a myth, and those persons who lately asserted this at St. Petersburg forget that mythology and the telegraph are incompatible.

I am a reality although only an ordinary mortal belonging to this nineteenth century, the past seventy years.

My native place is Bologna; formerly I only quitted it to travel, I was there in the times of universal enthusiasm in

---

* The Book of Job is one of the literary masterpieces of all time, and provides a profound discussion on the suffering of a just man. The date of the book is unknown. Job was called a righteous man by prophet Ezekiel, along with Noah and Daniel. See: http://biblescripture.net/Job.html

1847[1], I filled there several public offices, I have been occupied in state affairs, and have been honoured with a warrant of deputy in the Roman Parliament.

When I understood that I might be in the way of men of different political views, having myself only one faith and one word, and not having attached myself to any party, I resigned of my own accord a position of some importance and retired into private life.

From the obscurity of my retreat I followed political events, without forgetting the respect due to men, to the law, and above all to morality. Up to this period I had never dreamt of practising medicine; this however was the mission reserved for the remaining years of my life. I have commenced late; nevertheless the result which I saw during twenty years justifies me in thinking that I have achieved a revolution in medicine. I beneath to the world not a system of medicine, but the medicine which after twenty-five centuries was yet to be sought for. For a long period I had well known the emptiness of all the systems which every century and nearly every school had engrafted on the old trunk of the decayed tree of medical science.

My native country has always produced illustrious men especially in the medical sciences. Without being myself a doctor, I could easily understand that the medicine of the schools is powerless to cure the least malady although making

1. referring to the period when Pope Pius announced several progressive policies such as the promotion of railways, of gas-lighting, of an Agricultural Institute, and of some form of lay consultation in the administration of the States of the Church, on July 5th, 1847 the Pope granted a civic guard to Rome, and promised one to the provincial regions of the states of the church, all of which lent credibility, in many people's eyes, to the wider political authority of his papacy. (see: Italy in the Making , Vol. II By G. F. H. Berkeley, Cambridge University Press, 1936)

a parade of a great deal of science. I was acquainted with the celebrities of the Faculty of Bologna, doctors before whom the world bows, and myself also; for who does not appreciate these studies, this knowledge, and above all this tact which knows how to grasp in an instant the pathological condition of an or an, and which sees the slightest alteration concealed in an intestine? I saw doctors tell the patient: You have a lesion at two thirds of the third lobe, not a line higher nor lower. You have the lung attacked, the disease is under the tip of my finger, etc., etc.

These doctors were never deceived; after death the post-mortem examination showed the correctness of their statements. This was mathematical, but the patients died also mathematically.

The general opinion is, that it is the essential point of the practice of medicine to recognize exactly the disease; it is generally thought that the great number of patients who die under the hands of doctors, a number that Stahal[1] has estimated at seven in ten, have reason to complain only of ignorance or mistake. Here it was not a question of mistake, science was not in fault; in point of exactness, the diagnosis could not be more sure nor more precise; that which was wanting, that which did not preoccupy our doctors, was the cure; science pronounces certain maladies immovable, and that's all to be said about it.

Now I said to myself: what is the practice of medicine if it does not cure ? I understand that there are complaints that one cannot be conjure away[2]; I understand that every disease, arrived at a certain stage, only ends with the grave which awaits all mortals.

---

1. census records
2. vanished away through magic

But so many patients, banished by science as incurables and sent to be cured beyond the grave, seemed to me too numerous; I even regretted so much knowledge, so much genius expended to obtain such a feeble result.

Now what are the diseases cured by medical science? In following closely the results of the practice I found only too exact the statement I had read in Broussais,[1] namely, that: The science of medicine is the art of soothing the side with vain hopes; I succeeded in convincing myself that the greatest physician could not even cure a chilblain ; he could only anoint or cauterise the sore, but he did not destroy the germ of this disease which is in the blood, and is the same that, in a more advanced stage, gives rise to cancerous complaints.

The inability of the allopathic treatment, I like to repeat it, does not depend in general on want of knowledge; as far as concerns pathology, physiology, and anatomy, the human frame has con the subject of so many researches that there remains very little to examine ; the dissecting knife and the microscope have allowed research to be pushed to the rudimentary cells, I may say to the atomes[2] of the cell; by this powerful means of observation science is enabled to grasp the arrangements of the organs, their roles, their intimate functions, and to follow the phenomena of life to its last limit where commences the quid divinum of Hippocrates[3], the mystery of life.

But all this, proclaims Professor Peter, whose beautiful maxims I like to recall, is not the practice of medicine. The

1. in Paris, France

2. Number of Atoms in a Human Cell: Estimates range from 10 trillion to 100 trillion atoms. A cell contains elements such as, water molecules- atoms of hydrogen and oxygen. DNA is made up of atoms of carbon, hydrogen, and oxygen.

3. mysterious influence of the planetary bodies on humans.

doctor, said he, is not a simple practitioner. He ought also to be a man of science; but the science of the doctor is not simply chemistry, physics, and mechanics which are to him merely auxiliaries. The science of medicine is above chemistry and physics; it is the art of curing. I am going to put forth a paradox: It is necessary that the doctor should not only think of visiting patients but that he should think of curing them. Skepticism[1] in the therapeutics is a misdeed, because the skeptical practitioner does not act when he ought, or acts at hazard and without conviction.

The practice of medicine cannot be but medical science; this is what is said, this is what is repeated without ceasing, but which has never been a fact. Because in the mind of creators of systems, especially those so much brought forward in our days, medicine still remains medico-chemistry, medico-physics, or medico-mechanism. Actual therapeutics are confined to topical treatments, stopping short at the morbid symptoms which they keep off only by palliatives and being thus rendered powerless to prevent a relapse or a return of the disease - on the contrary, it is necessary to act on the organism in such a manner as to put it in a state to bring back, if possible, the affected parts to their normal condition.

This is why skepticism, I say, is a crime from the moment that it turns aside medicine from its aim, from its mission, which is, not to display a quantity of science, but to cure the greatest possible number of patients.

In the greater part of the treatises on medicine which come to us from Germany, there is a great luxury of anatomical and pathological details, but when you turn to the therapeutics they are cut short and despatched in a few pages. Thus, according to the celebrated professor of internal pathology,

---

1. the doctrine that true knowledge or knowledge in a particular area is uncertain.

that which is called medical science is chemistry, physics, anatomy, in a word natural history, rather than medicine; the accessory hides the principal. This scientific cloak has only served, for the greater part of the time, to turn medicine from its real aim, that is to cure the sick, prevent the returns and relapses instead of stopping at local applications and palliatives.

Finally, science is given to us in the place of medicine. Here are truths known to all the world, avowed by sincere practitioners, who nevertheless act as skeptics and believe their task finished when they have said : Your complaint is there ; such an organ is attacked at this point. These persons seem to forget that the patient requires a doctor to cure him: on the contrary they think they are paid to tell him : Science is not occupied in curing you, it has, in its infalliability,[1] pronounced you incurable.

Twenty years ago these reflexions tormented my mind. Boerhaave[2] said : "If one weighs attentively the good which a handful of true sons of Aesculapius has procured for men, and the evil that the immense number of doctors, from the beginning of the science even to this day, has caused to the human race, one will think without doubt that it would have been more advantageous if there never had been any doctors in the world."

Stahal would have wished "that a bold hand undertook to cleanse this stable of Augeas[3] : . . . . this science filled with

1. the inability to be wrong or conclusive.
2. in 1724, he first described the spontaneous rupture of the esophagus which typically occurs after forceful vomiting. A very uncommon, life-threatening surgical emergency.
3. Augeas, the mythical king of Elis, kept great stables that held 3,000 oxen and had not been cleaned for thirty years, until Hercules was assigned the job. Hercules accomplished this task by causing two rivers to run through the stables.

errors, in which the language is as defective as the thought, wherein everything is to be re-cast, both the principles and the matter."

Modern authorities are neither less numerous nor less unanimous in deploring the state of medicine, in denouncing the anarchy and the confusion that prevails "Complete absence of scientific doctrines in medicine; absence of principles in the application of the art ; empiricism everywhere : that is the state of medicine." (quote from: Joseph-François Malgaigne, French Surgeon and Medical Historian).

After this, how does it happen that the Faculties of our old Europe still crown doctors? How does it happen that the legislation of the most civilized countries surrounds with guaranties a profession, the chief masters of which would see it swept out of the world by a bold hand? What reason have these privileged bodies which have nothing but the rigid to kill without responsibility before the law, when their chiefs are the first to tell you, that "each name of a class of remedies, each formula even is an error" (quote from: Léon Louis Rostan, French Internist and a Member of the Académie Nationale de Médecine, Paris, France); that "the practice of medicine is not, in some respects, that of a reasonable man ;" that, "of all the sciences, medical science is the one which best depicts the aberrations of the human mind." Let us at least save these millions charged to the Budget of the state for professorships, laboratories, collections, etc., which have the name of medicine without the reality, for along while reform has been called for, but no reform is possible, until the true medicine, capable of curing, will be discovered. The erroneous system of Ptolemy would still prevail in astronomy if Copernicus and Johannes Kepler had not explained the movements of the stars by the true laws of nature: to depose the medicine of palliatives it is necessary to have found the medicine which cures.

This Hahnemann had already understood.

I have read or heard that this illustrious physician abandoned the usual practice of medicine, leaving a large and lucrative connection, because he had no faith in his science, after that he devoted his entire life to the research of means capable of curing, the complete absence of which had inspired him with disgust and aversion to allopathy.

Hahnemann divesting himself of the medical science drawn from schools followed experiments only; experiences alone made him discover "the law of similars" which has given the name to his doctrine.

I did not ignore the traditional custom of the academicians, always immobile, always looking back to the past, ready to attack any innovations; this is more especially seen in medical science, of which the doctrine of Hahnemann ought to have appeared as the negation, as he destroyed all systems imagined up to that time, by substituting for the ancient pathology a therapeutic purely symptomatic. This was certainly undermining all medicine which, with the exception of a mass of hypotheses and nosological studies[1], contains nothing that merits the title of medical science.

Adversaries could not now be wanting to the bold innovator; they appeared in troops, but were wrong in rejecting a priori[2], without examination, the doctrines of Hahnemann, and it happened that, in spite of his profound knowledge, in spite of his incontestable[3] genius in medicine, he could not escape the ridicule and sarcasm of his enemies, who fastening on the weak part, the form rather than the substance of the new doctrine, gained an easy victory in the eyes of the vulgar and superficial persons who are the great majority in all times and places.

---

1. a comparison among competing classification of diseases.
2. relating to reasoning or knowledge which proceeds from theoretical principle rather than from observation or experience.
3. undisputed or unquestionable.

But grave and enlightened minds judge differently; scientific men, such as Pidoux and Trousseau[1] did not disdain to take knowledge of all that is precious in homeopathy to enrich their therapeutics. In the work of Hahnemann there are two points to consider: the fundamental principle and the therapeutic method which is deduced from it. The homeopathic axiom or the law by which medicine acts in reason of its similarity with the morbid principles existing in the organism is as ancient as the time of Galen, who made it the scientific basis of medicine, and whose theory, developed by the learned Arabs, passed under a much more general form into the schools of the middle ages.

The following is found in Jean de St. Amands, a celebrated author of the 13th century: "according to Galen in his 4th book on simples, a veneno liberantes attrahunt per simile." Vomitus vomitu curator[2], is also an aphorism[3] of Hippocrates.

It is astonishing that only a simple novelty was seen in the principle proclaimed by Samuel who has simply defined and better applied the law of similars; it is more surprising that this law appeared strange to physicians when inoculation was already known. Vaccination, although introduced by charlatans, by an old woman of Thessaly, was finally adopted and practiced everywhere by physicians.

Besides this, in the first trials of inoculation, the learned doctors of Oxford found that a minute pellicule of the postule introduced into the nostrils of the patient produced effects too dangerous. Thus the principle and law of homeopathy was discovered two centuries before the time of Samuel, but the physicians accustomed to revolve in the vicious circle of

---

1. Georges Phillipe Trousseau (1833 –1894) and Hermann Pidoux (1808-1882),of France, authors of Treatise On Therapeutics.

2. Vomiting is managed by vomiting

3. spoken or written in a concise and memorable form.

hypotheses did not follow experimental induction and the natural logic of facts.

The Hahnemann therapeutic method comprises also the homeopathic pharmacodynamics or doctrine of doses. This point especially exercisedthe wit of his adversaries and gave rise to a storm of famous calculations, demonstrating, after their fashion, the emptiness of homeopathy. But the dosological questions are after all only questions of the necessary and sufficient quantity to produce a given effect.

Experiment alone can answer these questions, and it is known that Hahnemann was lead to the homeopathic dilutions by experiment. The celebrated mathematician Arago and his calculations should have been left in peace and the diluted remedies should have been proved by experiment without effect.

By this I do not wish to follow the disciples of Samuel as regards the question of their theories of dynamisation. I will only make a few remarks. In the first place it is necessary to distinguish two classes of action in matter, the massive action and the atomic action. The first follows (according to the immortal Newton) the direct ratio and the second, the inverse ratio of the masses themselves. Physics and chemistry, everywhere point out this double kind of phenomena. It is known that the atomic forces come into play when matter is disengaged from its massive aggregations in which this force exists in a latent state.

The effect of medicines analogous to massive or attenuated doses must therefore naturally be very different; a strong allopathic dose produces a sensible and visible action, which is not precisely a normal effect of the forces of the organism; for example, vomiting produced by Tartar Emetic. Experience, on the other hand, shows that attenuated doses change the actual state of the organism, arrest vomiting, spasms, fever, etc. These results obtained by means of homeopathic doses are not less real, less evident; hence it may be said, that the organism, under the influence of attenuated medicines, reacts by its proper force to disengage itself from an abnormal state, or from the morbid principles which produce such a condition. The allopaths, with their massive doses, obtain effects of a certain class; the homeopaths with their minute ones, procure results of a different order. It remains to be seen what are the effects proposed to be obtained to restore health, or in short to cure, because allopathy does not cure, this is known, this is admitted by all physicians of good faith.

The most important, in the colossal work of Hahnemann, is the profound study of the elective action of medicines, a study hardly commenced before his time, and which he advanced more than all his predecessors together. It is true that all the world has pretended to examine the action of drugs, from Hippocrates down to our times, and what has been the result of so much labor ?

Medicine has gained only three remedies, which in some respects, merit the name of specifies; these are mercury, sulphur, and Peruvian Bark. And again these specifics were not discovered by learned physicians; they were acquired by the vulgar, by quacks, in spite of the efforts of the doctors who pushed them aside; this is a matter of history. The rest is this confused mass, where are so well depicted the aberrations of the human mind; it is this arsenal of things called astringents, laxatives, sedatives, tonics, etc., where each formula is an error; what is more, the same drug is employed by two doctors as an astringent or a laxative, or tonic, or sedative, the unchangeable virtue of the substance having to lend itself to theory in fashion ; as we have before said, remedies have always been invented to conform to preconceived theories, without having first studied the true, natural and unchangeable properties of the medicinal agents.

If Hahnemann had only been the restorer of this study, he would have merited in this respect alone, the title of a great man, of an eminent reformer. He has also taught us to select the active principles in pharmaceutical materials, to separate the inert, heterogenous particles which are only a useless mass, to refine the materials employed in medicine and to condense the maximum of power in the minimum of mass. Thus prepared, the remedy acts directly on the organism and there displays all its powers, without passing through the changes which the massive doses undergo in the process of digestion.

For all this (I return to the meditations of twenty years since) it appears to me that the method of Samuel is much more than medical science esteems it, for I said the essence of medicine is the art to cure; allopathic medicine does not cure, it only dreams of making learned nosographies, but the means of conjuring diseases it does not possess, it does not seek them, and confines itself to proclaim the evils of man incurable instead of admitting its own inability.

This fearful train of incurable evils did not appear to me reconcilable with the idea of a providential order here below, nor worthy of the infinite wisdom, which has created the tree of good at the side of the tree of evil, and which in a word, has placed every thing in the world that is necessary to save it let it be either morally or physically.

The brute after its instinct goes to browse on the herb that cures him; man has more than instinct; intelligence is the guide which should suffice to sustain his existence.

I thought then of the first physicians who only employed herbs. The medicine of Hippocrates which, after so much progress and so many discoveries, is justly regretted in our day, was almost ignorant of this confused mass of materials which compose our collections decorated with the name of Pharmacopoeia. It is from the vegetable that the nourishment comes to the animals, it is by the vegetable that the world of animated beings is united to the inorganic creation. It is there also, I said to myself, that God has placed medicine.

With such reflexions I gave myself up to the research of something which could cure; thought to myself, that this something, still unknown, is not far from us; these active and powerful principles, proper for our cure, should be found prepared and ready made in the vegetable species.

I did not deceive myself. It soon happened to me to put my hands upon plants, the active principles of which, when extracted, produced cures. When I saw these effects repeated, always the same and never contradict, I said, there is the medicine. The diseases 011 which I made my first trials belonged to the scrofulous type, that is to say, alterations in the lymphatic system; this is why I called my first remedy by the word antiscrofoloso.

After that I carried my attention to the form and species of the diseases which this first remedy was fit to cure; soon the constancy of the effects and the habit of observation allowed me to insure the result in advance. I could no longer hesitate as the effects were certain in all varieties of scrofulous disease. These effects were wonderfully quick in the simple cases; the far advanced complaints diminished at first and then disappeared after a more or less long treatment, and the conquered diseases did not reappear.

Now what could be this plant? Could it be the universal panacea? In my inexperience, at first, I thought so. I was one moment on the point of admitting the theory of cancroides*

* diffusion theory of insect respiration ; in most spiders and scorpions, the respiratory gases are transported from tissues by circulating haemolymph to the epithelium of the book lungs where 0_2 enters and CO_2 leaves the body. This type of respiration shows certain physiological, though not chemical, analogies with respiration of large, vertebrate animals (Strazny & Perry, 1987).

which during a time has been considered as the cause of all diseases.

Time and experience showed me that the antiscrofoloso did not always produce, nor in all cases, the same good effects; the patients of sanguine temperament, plethoric, suffering from palpitations, hemorrhage, congestions, etc, were not cured under the influence of antiscrofoloso; this made me think that the blood is affected by more than one principle and consequently could not be cured by a single remedy.

But a second remedy which I at first thought to be also an antiscrofulous, gave me excellent results in all disorders of the blood properly so called, and in all disorders of the system of circulation.

For example an ophthalmic incurable by the first antiscrofolous yielded easily to the remedy which I believed to be a second one; this also made a wonderful cure of varicose veins. I saw the blood vessels, when enfeebled and wasted, rapidly reconstituated by this second antiscrofulous while the first produced no effect on them. I concluded from this that instead of being an antiscrofulous, my second remedy was an antiangioitico, and that if the first cured lymphatic diseases, the second removed all the alterations due to a vitiation of the blood.

As I have been able to subdue thousands of lymphatic diseases of every possible form with the antiscrofulo: as I have cured an infinite multitude of disorders of the blood vessels with the antiangioitico: it became for me an axiom (an axiom founded on facts always identical and observed daily during many years) that the antiscrofulo is the sure remedy for the lymph, as the antiangioitico is the sure remedy for the blood and that the causes of all our maladies are reduced to two only.

But the human organization presents differences everywhere; the "receptivity" of individuals varies infinitely according to age, constitution, sex, habits and the influence of the surroundings.

Hence the different forms and the complications of disease although all connected with the same two causes: alteration of the lymph and alteration of the blood.

Finally I have seen cases in which neither of the first two remedies effected a cure, whereas the employment of the two alternately carried off the victory. I conclude that the violation of the lymph brings on that of the blood and vice versa, and that there are mixed diseases requiring the simultaneous employment of the antiscrofoloso and the antiangioitico.

Henceforth I found myself in possession of fundamental facts; it was only necessary to extend researches in following the principle that every disease has its origin either in the vitiation of the blood or of the lymph or in a combination of the two. The same inspiration which led me to discover the antiscrofoloso and the antiangtoitico put me upon the traces of other remedies for diseases already developed, provided, let it be understood, that they had not already destroyed the patient, in which case it would no longer be a remedy that was required, but a miracle.

This is how the new materia medica has been formed which I at first demonstrated by innumerable cures and then announced to the whole world in pamphlets. Important publications have been put forth both in Italy and other countries, by physicians and honorable men, won over to the new science which possesses already a history, a bibliography in nearly all the European languages, a bibliography which I have completed in regard to the number of the remedies and especially the different modes of their application, so that every man may be his own physician, by the Italian edition of Elettromiopatia, scienza nuova, che cura il sangue e sana l'organtsmo. Casale-Monferrato, Paolo Berte'ro, tipo grafo editore, 1878[1].

To cure diseases hitherto regarded as incurable, this is indeed a revolution in medicine. The cures are thoroughly radical, as the complaints do not reappear. Under the influence of these specifics the organism is purified and visibly regenerated; in proportion as the remedies penetrate the body, the general nutrition assumes a regular progress, the cachexy disappears, a fresh complexion is visible, the tissnes acquire solidity and volume, and the wasted parts are themselves rebuilt.

In the presence of such remarkable facts, constantly observed everywhere and under very various conditions, I think it is permitted to lay down the principles of the new science. But, note well, I have not discovered a new system of medicine, but the medicine itself. All the systems have taken a false course. Why? Because they have searched for remedies after an order of preconceived ideas, and to conform to a theory established before hand, instead of commencing by experimenting on the materia mediea and making the theory after wards. This is what I have done, and which I wish to be remarked.

When I saw a vegetable substance curing herpes, I said: here is an antiherpetique[2]; when I saw the same remedy curing the gout, caries, coxalgia, etc., I pronounced it an antiscrofulous remedy. When under its action, I have seen cured at the same time, and in the same patient, herpes, gout, and diseased eye, I said: it is a remedy that acts on the mass of the blood. When I have seen the piercing pains of cancer cease,

1. Referring to his Article 'Elettromiopatia del conte Cesare Mattei' published in scienza nuova che cura il sangue e sana l'organismo (1878).

2. which cures herpes zoster.

the tumour itself lessen, become detached, and disappear; when I have seen with surprise the disorganized parts reorganized, I said: these remedies act on the entire organization. Finally when I have seen certain morbid affections disappear by simply touching them with certain liquids, and these liquids produce the effect of ordinary electricity, even the shock, perfectly astonished myself, I cried out: this is electricity.

I have seen all that I relate and have seen it now twenty years, and it is a sure fact that the diseases cured have never reappeared. These remedies, I said to myself, reach the evil in its very source and cure radically; It is the end of palliatives.

My discovery must not be placed side by side with the systems of medicine. If I lay down principles it is only to interpret facts; these nevertheless would equally exist, even if the interpretation is wrong, the remedies would lose nothing of their power; there would be nothing to change in the practice if it is found that I am deceived in my theory. The reader has already been able to grasp the theoretical principles of the new science, but I will resume them here.

1. The human organization is entirely composed 0t two elementary liquids, the lymph and the blood.
2. On the condition of these two liquids health and disease depend.
3. Every disease originates in a change either of the blood or of the lymph or of both at the same time.
4. Diseases which have the same remedy have a common origin, that is to say, they originate in a vitiation of the same principle, the lymph or the blood.

Hence it follows that all diseases curable by the antiscrofulous originate in a change in the lymph, as those which are subdued by the antiangioitico proceed from the alteration of the blood; finally maladies calling for the employment of these two remedies properly managed prove both parts of the organization affected.

5. It follows again from all that has been said that the form or localization of the disease is not sufficient for the selection of the specific remedies, it only serves to distinguish between lymphatic, angioitic, or mixed affections.

For example every skin disease can appear under a variety of different forms; yet the proper remedy would be found by ascertaining if the subject is lymphatic or sanguine.

Hence a diagnosis is extremely easy; if the pulse, the carotid arteries, the heart and the other symptoms indicate no defective state of the circulation of the blood, it is the lymph which is the only cause of disease.

At the Hospital of St. Theresa at Rome where, in two months, thousands of patients entered and were cured, I myself was able with some subordinate aid to make the diagnosis. Yet I was very seldomly deceived, as men of every class can testify, beginning with ambassadors down to simple workmen.

There, in the presence of the public, were accomplished amongst others, instantaneous cures, almost miraculous, and of which a German 'Medical celebrity, Docter Lutze, published a memoir at Leipsic. And as the details which I have since published were then unknown, it was an astonish ment, a stupefaction, an inexplicable mystery, yet it was the most simple thing in the world. It was a question of some herbs, of which some possessed the property of curing the lymph and others the blood, herbs which it had pleased God to put in my way when I was already advanced in years and had never made medicine my calling.

If now two remedies, two only, destroy the principles of disease, and if all diseases have only two origins, that is the lymph and the blood: which is the man, let him be ever so foolish, that cannot cure himself? Who cannot distinguish a skin disease from an inordinate palpitation of the heart? Who will confound a varicose vein with tetter[1]? Supposing one cannot distinguish that which everyone can discern, and the wrong remedy is used, no inconvenience can result from it, save only that the cure, contained in the true remedy, is wanting. This will be a sufficient warning and advice to take the other specific. It can not be too often repeated, all our diseases have their foundation in the lymph or the blood, in the white vessels or the red. All medicine is in this.

I say it is all in this, because no man in his senses would let a cancer develop itself, when he can so easily destroy the principle by curing the gland. No person would let himself be confined to the bed by the gout, sciatica, or pains in the head when with one of two remedies he can so easily eradicate the first symptoms.

Who would let himself he killed by cholera, when a few grains of antiscrofulous are sufficient to sweep out the germ as if by enchantment? Resist in the beginning, for any medicine will prove powerless after the sickness has gained full strength.

This all the world knows and understands: It is with such a simple theory and with such elementary remedies that every man can cure himself, and this medicine is certainly the medicine of the future.

I say the principles so simple, which serve as the base of the new medicine spring directly from experiment. The data of science come to their support; we shall see it.

Everyone knows that in the human body there are two sets of vessels charged to carry and distribute to all parts of the organism the nutritive fluids.

---

1. a skin disease in humans or animals causing itchy or pustular patches, such as eczema or ringworm.

The network of lymphatic vessels draws the whitish liquid called lymph towards the centre of circulation: in the red vessels, arteries and veins, circulate the blood properly so called, and which can be considered as elaborated and oxidised lymph. The discovery of the white vessels followed shortly after that of the circulation of the blood demonstrated by Harvey at the commencement of the 17th century (1628).

It is equally demonstrated that in space of time Varying according to individualities, all the integral parts of the tissues are more or less completely renewed. In fact the weight of a man after he has attained his complete development, remains stationary and does not change until the age when the decline of life commences. Yet however the body absorbs, during the period, every day a certain quantity of food, which by the process of nutrition is assimilated and added to the whole of the organs.

The invariability of the weight shows clearly that a quantity of matter, exactly equal to the weight of the elements drawn from the food, goes out or is eliminated from the body: the ingested material replacing the eliminated in equal quantities.

The fluid elaborated from the food, taken up by the chyle vessels[1], drawn by the lymphatic ducts mixes with the red blood, falls into the heart: from thence forced into the lungs, it becomes itself by oxidation red blood.

This blood, so to say, origin, spreads itself through out the organism, leaving everywhere new elements in its passage whilst the excess of oxygen contained in the blood burns up the old and worn out particles and converts them into products of elimination.

---

1. relating to any of numerous minute intestinal lymph-carrying vessels that convey chyle from the intestine to lymphatic circulation and thereby to the thoracic duct.

These products represented by water, carbonic acid, urea, etc., leave the frame by different issues, such as the skin, the respiratory organs, the kidneys, etc.

Thus the human frame is incessantly renewed by this admirably process of successive decomposition and recomposition, at the expense of the elements of the blood ; this is the first condition of our existence, of our life. In like manner, it is the relation either of quantity existing between the materials exchanged which constitutes the actual state of the frame, that is to say, health or disease. In purely chemical substitutions it is only the relation of weights which is considered. In the progress of biological phenomena there prevails an equivalence of a higher order, little known as yet, but which may be called organico-vital equivalence.

The normal state of health is the result of a certain number of forces distributed through all the organs of the frame according to a given law. From the brain to the fingers end all has a part to fill for the support of life; everywhere is work, and therefore consumption of force, or transformation of matter.

This is why the same matter cannot suffice indefinitely to support life ; matter which has been a certain time in the tissues, must be renewed; this matter has worked; work under whatsoever form it may be, is the result of its transformations; it is no longer capable of recommencing and travels already in the cycle of super-oxidation which tends to bring it back to the inorganic world. It is the steam which is escaping from the cylinder after having raised the piston, it is necessary to replace it by an equal quantity drawn from the source in order to recommence and continue the same work.

The normal continuation of the vital work is perfect health, which is itself the result of the balance between the force wasted and the force renewed.

Hence the elimination of exhausted matter represents the waste, whereas the assimilation of food is the restitution. Perfect health is thus found subordinate to the organico-vital equivalence of which we have spoken; that is to say, it is necessary that the atoms, which pass from the food by assimilation into the tissues, there deposit as much energy as the frame has lost in the work of elimination, by which living particles fall back into the inorganic world.

The state of perfect equilibrium in the organization, such as we have described, can only be purely ideal or could only have existed in man at the time of his creation. But it is necessary to remark that slight derangements in the accessory parts of a machine do not sensible derange the whole movement. There are in our body the essential organs of life and there are those that may be called accessory; life is threatened when the first are deranged; it is only troubled, and more or less painful, when the second are attacked.

We have borrowed these details from modern science to render more easily understood that life and health are in the blood and the lymph; that disease is in the alteration of the blood or the lymph, or of both together; that there are only two general and primitive causes of disease, and therefore two genera series of remedies, those which act on the lymph, which I call antiscrofulous, and those which purify the blood, which I name antiangioitic. By means of these remedies the constituent elements of all parts of the body are brought back to their normal condition; these elements by the work of their gradual substitution in all portions of the frame cause the exclusion of disease germs wherever they may be found. Hence it results that in purifying the blood, the action extends through the entire frame, thus destroying complaints. Hence again the reconstruction of wasted and partially destroyed tissues is no longer an impossibility. We have done it. This is the theory that I induced from the experiments; these are the principles by which I endeavour to account for certain facts produced by the new remedies. Scientific men may not only be contrary to my opinion, but may combat, reject and even ridicule my theoretical ideas, but they will be wrong in obstinately rejecting facts which remain incontestable.

After the preceding declaration, every man is at liberty to take hold either of the differences or the points of contact between the new science and homeopathy, properly so called, as founded by the illustrious Hahnemann. The one and the other rest on the law of similars, and in this respect my discovery is but the continuation and the crowning point of the medical science constituted by Hahnemann.

But with regard to the nature of the medicines, as well as the method of trying the power and mode of action on the organization, as well as certain theoretical points of view, there are between the two doctrines differences of such importance that it is necessary to indicate the same.

In the first place, Hahnemann stops at the morbid symptoms; he confines himself to combat the visible manifestations of the disease with his remedies, without tracing it back to its source and which consequently sooner or later is bound to reappear. We are speaking here, let it be understood, of serious diseases which invade the frame and threaten the source of life. By the homeopathic method these diseases cannot be radically cured; in this respect the homeopathic remedies, although more appropriate and applied more rationally, do not essentially differ from those of the old school, in fact do not go beyond the rank of palliatives. What is wanting in the Hahnemannian practice and which is its necessary completion, is exactly my discovery; The power which increases the action of medicines so much as to restore to the frame its lost vitality, repair its waste and deliver it from the morbid causes which give rise to different diseases. Add again to this the multitude of symptoms on which it is necessary to fix, according to the homeopathic system ; the variability of these, according to the differences proper to each organization, creates uncertainty, renders the diagnosis difficult, and the choice of the remedy embarrassing.

It is sufficient to open an homeopathic guide book to be convinced of this serious difficulty. At the side of each remedy are pathological tables mentioning a number of symptoms common to many of them: then it is necessary to distinguish and classify these symptoms in different orders and take into question their relative importance to grasp finally this or those which decide the choice. This is the cause that the practice of homeopathy is not so popular as is generally supposed.

All this is unnecessary for the application of the new materia medica; it is sufficient simply to decide between the lymphatic affections and the sanguine affections. It is rare that the subjects themselves do not show sufficient signs to distinguish one from the other. As for the remedies, the choice is generally easy. It is fixed so as not to be mistaken in- all special diseases requiring special remedies, such as febrifuges, expectorant, antisyphilitics, etc. in general the choice is between the antiscrofulous and the antiangioitics.

Simplicity is in everything the seat of truth, for the new science its simplicity is also its stamp and its demonstration, for every man can test the truth and the reality of its effects. This is what causes me to say, that the science I establish makes a revolution, and that it is certainly the medicine of the future. Its effects are prompt, frequently instantaneous; a few globules of antiscrofoloso given dry on the tongue stop a fainting fit, or a threatening of apoplexy. I have seen spasms of the womb relieved with the first spoonful of the solution of anticanceroso, a suspended labour re-established; the state of intoxication disappears in a few minutes by giving the globules of antiscrofoloso I have seen thousands of times acute throbbing pains, tetanic convulsions disappear by touching with my liquids, which in certain cases have produced a shock similar to that caused by a Leyden Jar[1], or the action of an interrupted current.

It is from these phenomena, which seem to me remarkable, that I have given the name- of Electro Homeopathy to the medicine which providence has made known to me. I wish to express by this word that these remedies, a class of electroides, conforming to the law of similars, possess a power and promptness which allows them to be compared to electricity.

It is from these new phenomena and especially from the changes that follow in the organism to bring about a state of health, that I say that my discovery is come to complete that which was wanting in the materia medica of Hahnemann.

Again a few words about another sort of difference between homeopathy and electro-homeopathy. Hahnemann tried the effects of his remedies on the healthy man; afterwards, from these observations he founded what the homeopaths call the pathogenesis of a medicine; this made known the sphere of action on the invalid. This rather indirect process leads to objections. Is it well ascertained that the effects of an agent remain identical whether applied to the healthy subject or the invalid?

This is not evident for all the world. On the other hand the pathogenetic tables are composed of symptoms verified and observed in many individuals for it will not be believed that this pathological train, which is found by the side of a remedy in an homeopathic manual, was met within a single individual, even if he should be a new job. Can it not be believed that the same remedy absorbed by two different organisms will not always produce identical effects? This appears to be plainly induced from my experiments; after this it seems difficult to guide oneself in

1. a device that stores static electricity between two electrodes on the inside and outside of a glass jar.

these symptomological tables and, above all, to specify what effect a given remedy will produce in many cases.

I thought there was only one way to go straight to the knowledge of medicinal power; that is to try the remedies on the sick man and to note the class of diseases it is adapted to cure. This way I have followed, a way free from every objection, from every difficulty; i cure the patient; there is a fact that cannot be contested; there also is the entire value of my medicine which ought to remain in the world, in spite of scientific chicancy preeminently[1] the positive medicine which does not require to be proved up by any theory, or which has for theory only the results of experiment under a general formula.

Hahnemann drew his materia medica from the three kingdoms of nature; his pharmacopeia contains mineral, vegetable and animal substances. The materia medica which I here make known is exclusively vegetable.

Finally the homeopaths, either to account for their infinitesimal doses, or to justify the employment of certain substances inert and without any medicinal action, have proposed mere empty explanations. Some went even so far as to believe that the mechanical processes of preparation, such as trituration, succussion, etc., developed a latent power in the substance; thus, in their language, the succussion and infinitesimal subdivision is called dynamisation. We have before said how much the purity of the medicinal substance and its subdivision, so as to render it absorbable by the organism, contribute to produce the effect. It is an old saying that corporanon aguntnisi solute[2]; and certainly the manner of preparing and bringing the remedy into contact with the organism is most important in a therapeutic point of view.

1. eminent above or before other medical systems.

2. the axiom that has been passed on from the days of alchemy.

But these are conditions which bring into play the forces of matter and it would be ridiculous to believe that these forces result from succussion and from the mechanical labor of manipulation.

I myself have no opinion of imaginary theories. I confine myself to evident facts and state that the general rule for my remedies is to place the dose in relation to the disease, that is to say, to diminish the dose in proportion to the gravity of the malady. By the word dose I understand that which it is agreed to call dilution.

The rule stated is drawn from experience, and even if the theoretical reason cannot be given, it would no less be the general canon of Electro-Homeopathy. During the first ears I administered one drop of essence in a large g ass of Water and I cured invalids by thousands; afterwards I reduced the remedies to form of globules and have since given, in ordinary cases, one globule dissolved in a glass of water to be taken by spoonful's within the 24 hours of the day; I descend to the second dilution, and in rarer cases to the third; on the other hand, in some cases, I go up to very strong doses[1]. Here are the facts which I point out, saying, at the same time, that the dose should be in inverse ratio to the gravity of the disease; I add that it is necessary to know, if required, how to employ the whole scale of dosology.

I do not go so far as to say that I dynamise matter; I have not the power which belongs only to the Creator qui effudit illam super ommia opera ejus[2], as it is written in the Book of Wisdom.

Instead of having recourse to occult qualities and imaginary theories, which should have been left to the alchemists, the

---

1. In the case of a Princess whose cure did not progress in employing 3 spoonfuls of white electricity in the bath, l ordered a half litre to be used ; the Princess came out cured of her chronic and serious infirmity.
2. he is with that includes everything works.

homeopaths should have placed the facts in a clear light and shown unbelievers that, from doses called homeopathic, real effects were obtained. The facts exist, although the method and reason cannot be accounted for, and facts, in medicine, count more than all the volumes of medical science that have been written since the origin of the art. But, in the case which occupies us, it appears to me that the theoretical reason, why the quantity of the remedy should be diminished when the disease is serious, can easily be found. In fact, what is a cure ? It is the result of organico-vital reactions caused by means of agents which we call remedies. These reactions are so much the less as there remains less vitality in the centre of the organism or that the disease is grave. Thus it is why, in my opinion, it is necessary to lessen the quantity of the medicine in ratio to the intensity of the malady. To do otherwise would be to ask more of the organism than it can perform; it would be contradicting the general law of nature, namely that the reaction is always Equal and opposed to the action.

Great pain, large remedy, the vulgar will exclaim without doubt. But the large remedy, I say, is not in the great mass of the medicine; it is simply the quantity necessary and sufficient to cure.

For example, when I have had to treat herpes, acne and many other skin diseases I have constantly remarked that, with the ordinary dose of the first or even second dilution, the complaint gradually disappeared, whereas the eruption increased with a dose of 10 globules, and became enormous when 40 or 50 were given daily. At this time similar results have been observed in the treatment of every class of disease. But it must not be forgotten that, the lower the dilution the more frequently must the doses be given, so that these infinitesimal quantities produce, by successive and increasing reactions, a definite result, the cure. See how, without being a doctor, I have discovered not only the materia medica but the methods and rules for its application.

Observation and experiment, how many things could they not teach us which, so often, pass by unseen! It is the education received, the direction imparted to our intelligence, in early life, which often prevents us forming a just opinion of facts which fall daily under our notice.

But we are early accustomed to routine, that is to say, only to repeat what others have said; science is spread before the eyes of our intelligence ready made; even the very words that are necessary to repeat to be instructed and learned are placed on our lips. Frequently at the bottom of these theories which cost us so much study there is the emptiness of human ignorance adroitly masked by conventional phrases. It is only by this routine that prejudices are perpetuated. It is thus that it is generally believed to be an absurd thing that medicine can exist outside of the Faculties, and that all are disposed to ridicule men who, outside of these learned bodies, announce to the world a discovery touching the sacred domain of the academy; and thus again supported by prejudices and ignorance the physicians have the right to kill us, and to forbid us to cure.

This is how our society is constituted and the human race submits to it.

I had hardly discovered the new therapeutic agents and collected sufficient results to convince one that my discovery was a grand one, certainly the most useful that had been made to this day, I felt it my duty to make it known and spread it abroad for the good of all men. I was going to claim neither money nor honor; I simply obeyed the dictates of humanity; I did not pretend to be believed in words. I commenced by facts, I made numerous cures. What was the reception of the physicians? I am about to relate it.

During ten years I held at Bologna public meetings where I received the refuse of hospitals in a crowd, all these unhappy objects to whom science had said its last word. The incurables were cured ; it was the power of St. Anthony, said the vulgar.

But the physicians, who had little faith in St. Anthony, came to assist at the consultations, took notes, one of them, Doctor C., kept a register with the names of the patient treated, all the details, and even the duration of the cure. After much pressure Doctor C. published a notice of the authentic cures. I began to believe that after this only electro-homeopathy would be practiced at Bologna. I was deceived : a demand was simply made to the Perfect to close my consulting rooms, and Bologna, the scientific town, continued to practice science and to allow the incurable to die very learnedly.

The miracles of St. Anthony, seen by the public in a celebrated city of a hundred thousand inhabitants, were noised abroad and spread throughout the whole Peninsula, for people came from all parts of Italy to my consultations; that what happened at Rome (where I was invited by that conscientious physician L. Pascucci) made known the marvels of electro-homeopathy to foreigners. At the hospital of Ste-Theresa at Rome I received in three months nearly 12,000 persons, from people of the highest rank, Italians and strangers down to a lad of the streets; every one saw clearly the reality and power of the new therapeutic agents. It was enthusiasm, it was stupefaction; the rooms, the stair-cases, the court yards swarmed with sick persons; it was necessary to place guards to keep order.

I only relate facts and this a small part relative to the history of electro-homeopathy. The press and the correspondence of so many persons spread it everywhere; amongst others the celebrated doctor Lutze published at Leipsic the account of a cure which seemed miraculous to him: a blind man brought into the operating room went away reading a book!

A new phase in the history of electro-homeopathy was about to commence. A number of doctors asked for the remedies to try themselves. Of course I did not refuse them; I supplied them a sufficient long time to enable these gentlemen to make all sorts of experiments. I was so certain of the effect, that I was not surprised when I heard of extraordinary cures, of which these good people took the trouble to inform me, and which some of them published accounts of, which they kindly addressed to me. My greatest astonishment was when, all at once, the doctors were quiet and ceased to inquire for the remedies. But they required now more than the remedies; now what? the Formula !

Yes, the formula, they wished to cure by the formula. For an instant I thought that the doctors in question had taken in their heads to practice medicine after the fashion of the physicians of Morocco, who treat wounds by the virtue of a verse of the Quran, written on a piece of paper and carefully applied to the part. But I was deceived, and this was the false argument that I made; I thought: these physicians have tried the remedies and are convinced of their efficacy; but as doctors only search and ask to be successful in the treatment of disease (it is their mission, their oath), therefore they beg for these remedies which cure.

Finally, information from beyond the seas, from the old world and the new, especially from correspondents at Leipsic and New York, came to enlighten me. I saw a new light, a radious verity[1], a reality, a discovery more positive, more convincing and less open to discussion than electro-homeopathy. But, in short? It was very simple: a globule was sold for a dollar at New York, and a German silver coin at Leipsic ; 800 francs was the price asked for one of my bottles of fluid. Then I understood the more logical and more scientific argument of these gentlemen; they said: we have cured cancer, gout, coxalgia, stone, etc., etc., with your remedies, which could, in our hands, be sold and produce three francs a globule;

1. eternal principles

therefore give us the formula. If it is refused to us, we shall do all in our power to annihilate your discovery, and proclaim everywhere that it is mere quackery. The remedies without the formula are only good to cure diseases; there is no worse disease than an empty pocket. Besides what shall we do, we, who have studied to live on illness, if this medicine of globules, of electric drops, should come to replace the official medicine, and the materia medica of our pharmacopoeia ?

These gentlemen had grasped all the importance of the medicine, of which they had proved the reality, and all that which would ha pen if it came to be spread abroad. They said: the new medicine is good; only it is necessary that it should not be sufficiently so, as to ruin the old; but, so that it should not cause a dangerous revolution, it must remain in the medical periphery and we ought to have the formula. The formula were demanded from all parts, for, wrote these physicians, we are afraid of secret remedies. I refrain from publishing a list of all these philanthrophists of different countries, whose correspondence I have preserved. At that time I answered to the most worthy by printed letters ; a number of these will be found in my Italian edition: *Elettromiopatia del conte Cesare Mattei*[1], Castle Monferrato. -Paolo Bertero, tipografo-editore, 1878. For the remainder see my little works: *Un poco di storia sui rimedi Mattei*, Bologna, Istituto tipografico[2], 1871, *Emancipazione dell'uomo dal medico pei rimedi Mattei*[3], Bologna, 1875.

To sum up: the medical question was to be transformed into a commercial one; these gentlemen understood it at once, but

1. Electrohomeopathic Medicines by Mattei (Indian edn: Originals).
2. A little bit of history on Mattei remedies, Bologna, typographic institute.
3. Liberation of the man from the doctor by Mattei remedies.

I, the author of the discovery never dreamt of it! There was in it, however, a large and good business; negotiations, offers and projects were not wanting; it was necessary to decide.

Between a personal benefit and a benefit, which I regard as sent from heaven for all men, I thought it better to give the medicine to the world than to increase my fortune. To insure this I have not given the formula to these philanthropists, because, after all, they have discovered nothing, and, on the other hand, they did not appear disposed, after what I have heard from Leipsic and New York, to render, peculiarly popular this medicine, which has been discovered for the poor as well as the rich. I could see, that, in the medical periphery, this medicine, instead of causing a revolution, and spoiling so many arts and professions, would be spoilt itself, and after having made some fortunes, would disappear from the world at the death of the inventor.

I have, therefore, kept the medicine which belongs to me, as I alone discovered it, at the price of my researches. Without calculating my expenses I reduced the tariff of Leipsic from a German silver coin to one hundredth of a franc although leaving to the dispensaries a five fold profit on the medicines bought at Bologna. This is how I came to resolve the question under its double aspect, medical and economic.

But it is a secret remedy, cried the vexed philanthropists! Yes, I answer; it is a secret which I intend to guard in my own hands as long as I have not insured the benefit of it to men: as long as I have not found sure and faithful hands to preserve it for the world, and persons sufficiently humane, not to convert it into a speculation, sufficiently honest to make an ordinary cure at the expense of a few centimes[1] daily, as I have regulated it myself. I understand, it will not be the medical periphery which will accept the medicine which cures. The doctors do not care for such remedies, but only for the formula.

1. a monetary unit equal to one hundredth of a franc.

The formula, during my life, I guard myself; after me do not fear the deluge! Everything is already arranged[1], everything insured so that this providential discovery is not lost, and that this revolution should be accomplished in the world.

---

* In 1895, Count Mattei, suspecting Sofia Condescu the Romanian wife of Mario Venturoli (adopted son of Mattei) attempting to kill him using a turkish cafe containing poison, hunting Mario Venturoli and his Romanian wife Sofia Condescu from the castle and disassociating them from his property by making Will in favor of his daughter Maria Bonaiuti for his all inheritance including his secret formulas. (see : Pharmacodynamics in Spagyric Medicine (Plant Alchemy) – by Dr. Debasish and Dr.Sudeshna Kundu, Edited by Gisela Bruckel, Germany, El Akrem Hayouni, Tunisia, Forwarded by Dr. Peter Morrell (UK), Prof.Luigi Vernacchia, Dr. Fabio Ambrosi, Italy (LBO Publishing, 700 N Valley St., Suite B PMB 11884 Anaheim, CA 92801, USA) for Mattei's Secret manufacturing process, and Mysticism, Romance & Secrets of Count Cesare Mattei by Dr. Debasish Kundu (LBO Publishing, 700 N Valley St., Suite B PMB 11884 Anaheim, CA 92801, USA) for Properly Transcripted Formulas of Count Cesare Mattei. In India both books are available with Originals, Delhi.

Mattei died at the age of 87 on 3rd of April 1896, while suffering from senile dementia, the unfortunate outcome of poor health in old age.

After Mattei's death the castle witnessed a bitter legal ramification over it's inheritance, and in 1904, Mario Venturoli, having opposed the Will hired top lawyers and bribed medical doctors providing a false medical report on the state of mind of the Count in his last phase of life, succeeds in proving that the Count was suffering from Alzeimer's and obtaining back much of the inheritance.

It was during this phase, production of Electrohomeopathic medicines was suffered in castle. The pre and post first World War scenario also contributed to the decline in the production and supply of the medicines.

Rejected by you, my medicine turned towards the people: "The people alone has the sentiment of the future and the intuition of truth. All the social creations of the past century proceed from it. It is by it that liberty has found and created the happiness of a gigantic nation beyond the Atlantic Ocean." (Mure) The people does not demand formula, it is not afraid of secrecy, it only wishes to cure; it has said in its common sense that health is the greatest treasure of the world. This people, there is a long time that it has been allowed to perish, although paying dearly the recognized formula of the official medicine, so that it cannot avoid trying my secret remedies which cost so little and yet CURE. But, you know, trial convinces even the physicians; here the results never fail, it is only necessary to say : Try it.

There are centuries that you make attempts with out curing ; the people commence to understand this, but it does not comprehend how men, certainly respectable to their knowledge and probity, as there are so many in the medical class, men who have devoted themselves incessantly to the study of medicine, who have sufficient self-denial to condemn themselves to tedious work in the pestiferous chambers of laboratories, to breath all their lives the surroundings of hospitals, and the miasma which exhales from the bed of the patient, running the risk of never having an hour's sleep free, and all this frequently for a recompense which is not in proportion to the sacrifice, the people does not understand that the men, who do all this that I have described, are not yet able to cure many complaints that the lower classes, the ignorant cure by means of secret remedies.

Here is the reason why the people does not inquire, like scientific men, about what you call my secret; it is because the people has been itself delivered by this secret from coxalgia, caries, cancer, staphyloma, elephantiasis, stone, gout, chronic bronchitis, and a thousand evils which you have never thought of relieving.

The people has seen this during ten years at Bologna, then at Rome, then everywhere, and continues to see it; it has also seen the physicians who assisted and who could see better; now the people is astonished that the doctors have not accepted this medicine with the secret of curing; the people has revolted against science, when it understood that science continued to amputate legs, which my remedies, tried in despair, have cured, and to kill, with opium, the patients declared incurable how would have left my rooms thoroughly cured. The people will make the revolution, a revolution not requiring arms, which will shed no blood, which overturns nothing, not even the medicine of palliatives, which will find itself overthrown by its want of power to withstand the medicine which cures. At this hour the revolution has commenced; electro-homeopathy is in Italy, in Germany, in Russia, in England; it will pass the Caucasus and will penetrate into India and Japan.

The effects produced by it have left profound traces; adepts have everywhere been made. But those who have recognized the truth have not always had the good faith and the courage to proclaim it. I could quote names here which became celebrated by cures made with my remedies in Italy and in foreign countries; these are prodigies, but these workers of miracles take care to disguise my globules in every way and to employ them secretly for fear of compromising their prestige. These however are the jokers who ask for the formula and fear the secret remedies of Bologna. Honest men have welcomed the truth, and openly rendered homage to it. Already, in 1869, the honest doctor L. Pascucci published at Rome an interesting account of electro-homeopathy to make known the wonders he had witnessed, an account which was soon translated into French, and several other languages. On his part Doctor C put forth in 1867 a detailed notice of the favorable results of the great experiments made at the public meetings in my palace at Bologna. The celebrated physician, Acwort, in 1870, published some extraordinary cures, in the English press, among others that of his wife, who by means of a few grains of antiscrofoloso recovered the use of her right arm, which she had lost a year previous.

Not less astonishing cures were reported in the Italian, English and German press, and Doctor Zimpel published (Leipsic 1869) an important work on the marvellous remedies of Count Mattei: Die Vegetabilische Elektrizität (German).

My first little book, un poco di storia sui rimedi Mattei (Bologna) 1871) was at once translated into German by Girtler at Vienna. L'emancipazione dell' uomo dal medico, which I published at Bologna in 1875 went through several editions, and translations into different languages, as well as the preceding work. Two works of Doctor Regard of Geneva appeared in 1872 to 1873, the first entitled, "Quelques mots sur les specifiques du Comte Mattei," the other : "Guide pratiqae pour l'emploi des du comte Mattei (Pfeffer et Puky, Geneva.)

M. Bérard Pastor at Loriol (Drome), from the indications which I supplied him and aided by my treatises, has edited guide books which have been translated into nearly every European language; not long ago a journal having for title, The Electro Homeopathic Review was founded at Geneva, for the diffusion, said the editors, of the new science, to announce especially the cures and the success of the new therapeutic agents.

It was to complete this bibliography and to publish that which was yet unknown, all the resources of the new medicine, that I published an Italian work, a long-time demanded by persons who had not or who did not wish to have doctors to treat them. This book was translated into Russian at St. Petersburg immediately after it appeared[1]. Finally it is to throw a complete and universal light on the subject that I am decided to put forth this new work and which I think necessary to have compiled in the most wide spread language, for the book is addressed, as my medicines are, to the entire world.

All this movement is produced and progresses every day in spite of the pretended secret; this proves that it is not necessary to reveal it to the first physician that comes along. As has been seen, very honorable doctors have welcomed and illustrated the new science by their publications; I could quote many others, physicians, scientific and illustrious men of all countries, who have not rejected the remedies, the mystery of which I defer to a latter period to divulge. These worthy people know that secrecy neither adds to nor detaches from the value of the remedies, which they take with more confidence than the well known drugs of ordinary medicine; they know well that I only guard the secret, for the present, to guarantee the purity of the remedies, to trust aside sophistication and the cupidity of those who only see in the greatest inventions: money and profit; they understand also that, at the present moment, my medicine would have been done for, if I had given the formula to all those who demanded it.

Respectable persons, although admitting the necessity I am under, of guarding the secret for the present, have shown their apprehension for the remedies after my death. Those who

1. A German translation of it was also issued, by thousands of copies at Stuttgart at the beginning of the year 1879. One copy was sent to me; it was quite accurate ; all the others sold in Germany contain false indications so as to recommend the remedies invented by Albert Sauter at Geneva and labelled with the same names as the real remedies of Bologna. I protest against those translators and their intrigues.

know the deceitful and untrustworthy struggle that I have sustained during twenty years, the persecutions, attempts even against my life, fear that crime or spite will finish by burying my discovery in my tomb.

I wish to assure them once more that this will never happen[1].

I should prefer that God, and especially men allow me to live all my days, but, whatever may happen, my remedies cannot be destroyed; everything is foreseen, everything arranged, a long time since, so, that at my death, my discovery, which I regard as a benefit. direct from heaven, remains to the world.

Why should one fear that I do not take sufficient precautions for it to survive me? I have laboured much to establish it, and I shall work more, during the days that remain to me, to insure MY LEGACY TO HUMANITY.

There are, also, worthy people who wish to see physicians at the head of electro-homeopathy. Physicians will always be welcome; I even say they will be the most welcome; as medical science is not opposed to this practice, my remedies will be only better applied by men who are acquainted with the structure of the organs and the morbid lesions. It is not necessary that I repeat here that it was to physicians that I made the first appeal, to whom I offered and gave my remedies gratis; neither is it necessary that I again testify my respect for the true sons of Aesculapius[2]. But the greater part do not want me; the greater part have rejected the new therapeutic

---

1. I repeat here that which has been so often said and which ought to suffice to dissipate the anxiety of M. Berard, or rather the anxiety that M. Berard seeks to cause. The threats and the tyrannical monopoly of which he speaks seriously in n° 8 of his Review.

2. Aesculapius was the god of medicine in ancient Greek religion and mythology.

agents, and I cannot convince these good only regard him and the staff of the doctors that these agents create no danger to their profession, if it is not to simplify their practice, and, what is more, to supply them with sure means to cure the greater part of the patients which, for the want of remedies, they are forced to let die. The greater number of physicians, even after having clearly seen it, said: No matter, they die legally. (Un poco di storia sui rimedi Mattei, p. 15, Bologna, 1871,) I answer that at present it is useless to wait to see the physicians come; but the time may come when they will be obliged to do so. After the history of twenty years I can say, that a spontaneous conversion, on their part, would be a greater miracle than the wonders of electro-homeopathy. I do not flatter myself to possess such powerful-specifies. But this miracle will be the effect of the whole, the last result of electro-homeopathy. I have reason to think so, as it has already happened so many times.

Against all changes, against all discoveries of new remedies, made outside the medical circle, doctors have always been seen to declare war.

Thus it was that learned medicine, for a long period, opposed the use of quinquina[1], brought from America by the profane, and this powerful febrifuge, known to the savages of Quito[2] for centuries, would not have triumphed in the struggle against Mohy, Chiffiet, Plemp, etc[3]., if it had not worked a great miracle; the cure of the Countess of Chincona, the wife of the Viceroy of Peru!

Thus it was again that physicians dreaded the inoculation of small-pox taught to Emmanuel Timoni, member of the

1. an aromatised wine, traditionally contains cinchona bark.
2. traditional practitioners of Ecuador.
3. See: Journal der Chirurgie Augen-Heilliimde, Berlin, 1827 available with Internet archive, https://archive.org

faculty of Padua and Oxford, by an old woman of Thessaly ; and it was by the miraculous effects, and the influence of Lady Montague who demonstrated them, that the medical College of London decided to make a trial, and then to adopt this prophylactic against a disease which ravaged Europe.

I am convinced that the same will happen to electro-homeopathy, which is not like these drugs, an isolated means, frequently powerless, a simple palliative of some diseases, but a complete medicine, certain, radical, applying especially to complaints hitherto pronounced incurable. I say that such is my conviction, based on the history of the past, and on facts accomplished during the past twenty years ; yet, after all, I think that it is the reality, the truth of a discovery which best insures his triumph. In the combat it is not truth which falls ; it there purifies itself to shine more brilliant after, and casts off, in the struggle, the veil of error, even as the sun frees itself from the fogs of the horizon, to lighten with a pure light the eyes even of those who fly from it. Let us see if prejudices, opposition, controversies have been able to stifle the discoveries which, since the 16th century, have come, in turns to upset the ancient scientific edifice and to shake the secular authority of the Academies. The men who were the first to announce new truths, were branded ; but Galileo on his knees, Fulton ridiculed, are trophies that lasted only a day for their enemies, but which, on the morrow, became titles of glory for their names; and the conquered Academy raises their busts after having rejected them! Electro-homeopathy is already known; it only requires to be widely spread to take that place to which it is called by its nature and importance ; it will bring about a beneficial reform in medicine. This reform may be a long time before being thoroughly accomplished, but it cannot fail: that which relieves so much misery interests every one.

There are reforms which start from the summit of society, and- there are those which ascend from the base to gain the summit. It is this ascending progress, which we have observed for a-century, which grasps best the questions which concern it, which first came out of the middle ages, which stripped legislation of the rubbish of the past. The people is not the lowest of men; neither is it a class of society ; it is society, the body and mind of the nation. When governments do not include the people in question which concern it the most, they march in a road, closed at the end.

It is thought that medical reform can only be the work of governments; this is a mistake, or, at least, there is a distinction to be made here.

Medical affairs are subject to special laws, amongst modern nations. It is the same as regards the practice of what is called: official medicine. Among the Greeks, the Romans and the Arabs, the physician did not hold his mission from the state; he did not go to be crowned with the academic laurel; the law accorded no diploma to authorize him ; he put him self forward, simply, at his own risk and peril; he formed his connection by his means and especially by his talents. In the first centuries of our era medicine was practiced, in this way by the monks and the Church, up till nearly the 13th century, when the Popes interdicted the practice of medicine to the clergy. The physicians, in this period, were learned encyclopedists, and filled one of the most remarkable parts in the governments of the epoch.

The Popes organized the Faculties amidst which shone Medicine. These were learned corporations which delivered diplomas and patents, after a course of study and public examinations, giving faculty to - practice medicine.

The candidates took an oath, at the time of reception, on the works of Hippocrates and Galen. The Faculties, not only gave the power to practice, but placed the licenciates under their protection, outside of the common laws ; for these corporations were themselves independent, and possessed their arms, their militia and their banner. By degrees, as civilization, urged by the powerful breath of the people, made its way, these privileges fell, legislation stripped of a quantity of old customs, tended, without ceasing, to realize the principle of the equality of all men before the law, claimed by the people. Equality before the law, I say it openly, is not the social level of the communists, nor the unnatural dream of the socialists; it is sin is justice among men, proclaimed by the Gospel of Christ[1].

It will be thought that I go straight to the conclusion: that the privileges and guarantees, which the law has continued to grant to Faculties and to the medical profession are relics of the middle ages which ought to be abolished by popular action. God forbid! nothing of this ought to be said or done; nothing of this is necessary to reform the practice of medicine. Let the Faculties continue to grant diplomas, and the Academies to unite and concentrate all the means for the progress of medical science; science is truth; nothing but blasphemy and stupidity can despise it: Sapientiam et doctrinam stalti despictunt[2].

Could the people be told that it ought henceforth to abandon study, to no longer think to maintain the sacred fire on the altar of Minerva, in order to carry always higher the torch of science in all the branches of human knowledge? what would become of a nation which would forget, for a moment, the study of sciences which form its most glorious title to fame, and which decree the rank that it occupies in the scale of civilization? And, in the number of the most elevated sciences, those which treat of life, the human organism and its functions must well be included. I repeat, with the professor of internal pathology at

1. news of the coming of the Kingdom of God (Mark 1:14-15)
2. senseless foolish, stupid ones acting without reflection or intelligence!

the University of Paris: it is necessary that the physician should be a scientific man; it is not the scientific man who can deny the new truths that I proclaim.

Among the injuries that have been hurled against me, after the publication of my Italian book, is this: that I reach ignorance and obscurity, that I even pretend to demolish the colossal edifice[1], built up from Hippocrates to our own time! These men attack me, in the name of science, and only find abuse to refute me with ! they have not refuted me, for an insult is not an answer.

For the rest, I have sufficiently explained myself with these critics, with regard to what they call medical science, not to dwell on it any longer, see my italian pamphlet: La scienza nuooa dd come Cesare Mattei—E smkmza 'vecchia del dottore 0., chez P. Bertero, Casalc Monferrato, 1878.

What then is the reform of which you speak, will be asked now? What ought to be done so that your newly found medicine can be established ? As regards the Faculties and the physicians, I answer: there is nothing to be done; respect them and leave them as they are.

But the law protects their position, gives them the right to regulate the practice of medicine, consequently to repel you, to interdict you and your remedies; this is nothing; I am about to explain it.

The law, equal for every one, cannot maintain privileges for any class or any profession. It would be necessary to go back, some centuries, to find laws of this class, to go into China to still find castes organized by the state. Thus, what you think in our countries, are privileges for the physicians, are, partly, guarantees for the people, for it is not the profession of doctor

1. Another famous temple, the colossal edifice known as the Olympieum, lay at some distance from the Acropolis on the southeast of Greek & Roman Mythology.

which the modern legislator places under the patronage of law; it is the health of the people, the life of its subjects which is of supreme interest to every government. This, with out deception, is the reason why our civilized governments decree for the medical profession and materials; this is just.

This is just as long as it regards official medicine ; here the intervention of the state is necessary to regulate, either the material, dangerous in its nature, or the action, the guarantees of capacity, even the studies and the degree of knowledge of those who are called to use it in their official profession.

Let, now, the first comer practice medicine with therapeutic agents, containing life or death, or rather death close to life; deliver these poisonous drugs to inexperienced hands. The earth, then, could still conceal the errors of these newly arrived doctors ?

It is, I say, to warn off or diminish the accidents of this kind, that the law inspects the materia medica and that there are commissions of hygiene to approve of medicines before delivering them to circulation.

As to the profession, it is evident that the State has the right to impose regulations, programmes, courses on all those who come to claim, from it, a title assuring a social position. And, besides, medicine, such as our Faculties have made it, (as Professor Peter has said very much to the point) is science, chemistry, physics, physiology, etc., much more than it is medicine.

Take away these sciences, there remains nothing which can be called official medicine. See, now, that in default of medicine, the accessory sciences must, of necessity, be preserved and, therefore: the organized Faculties, the laboratories, the courses, the diplomas, in fact all the scaffolding of the official medicine.

To sum up, this medicine is, from its nature, and under all reports, subject to the law; and, not only would the public health be endangered, but the very existence of medicine itself the day when the State should leave it entirely free.

Nothing of this, that we have remarked, applies to any medicine, free from danger, which requires no diploma, and can be practised, with the aid of elementary knowledge, by every man who has a slight habit of observation. Such a medicine is, by its nature, free in all States of the world, it is by natural right,—the State cannot restrain it without violating personal liberty, the most sacred of all.

It is, now, understood what is the medical reform that I await, and which cannot fail to arrive. It is a very peaceful reform, as there is nothing to change, either in the official medicine or in the laws; the laws will continue to regulate dangerous drugs and large doses, but the globules which the doctors, by mockery, call innocent grains, afford no matter to the laws; my doctors, who do not incur the risk of killing, who do not go to demand diplomas, do not issue from a Faculty; for, if the physician could better show off the wonders of Electro-homeopathy, these wonders could take place, equally, without being a learned man. As long as I thought that all physicians only sought the means of cure, I addressed myself to them ; I left them a long time to experiment thoroughly. When I well understood what the majority wanted, I addressed myself to the profane; I made an appeal to the people; I commenced by publishing a first popular little work (Un poco di storia sui remedi Mattei) to denounce the conduct and the bad faith of certain doctors, then I published another pamphlet (Emancipazione dell' uomo dal medico pei Rimedi Mattei) ; then I furnished to persons, who came to offer their services for the propaganda, materials for guide books; the books appeared and are spread, every where, in many languages ; persons, who had never practised medicine, treated themselves and taught others. Finally, when I saw that it was necessary to place myself at the head of the movement, I finished the work commenced by the adopts; I published the guide book, in which I laid forth all the resources that can be drawn .from electro-homeopathy for the good of the people, which the greater part of the doctors, refuse to treat by this powerful means.

My discovery is now handed over to the people; it spreads and will spread more and more.

One day, the people will say to the physicians: you are the deputies, the mandatories of society to watch over our maladies and to cure us; the laws recognize you as the public officers of health. You do not cure us, you say that we ought to die, if we are attacked by cancer, consumption, gout, stone, cholera, etc., but we see that these diseases can be cured. Only, the doctors refuse to employ these excellent remedies, because they are secrets, discovered by a man who is not a doctor of your medical science. You have a thousand reasons, doctors! but, we no longer want you; we demand, in the name of the law, which protects the health of the people, that every doctor, who, being able to cure us, leaves us to die by palliatives, be responsible to society; for, on your part, leaving us to die, when we are curable, is a crime.

Behold the reform accomplished without noise, without action of any sort. When the people will have understood this, statesmen will see what is necessary to do to revise the legislation.

The partisans of Malthus may be alarmed at a luxury of vitality, the exuberance of which would impede the march of their politics ; but it is probable, that the most enlightened governments will be the principal to assure this powerful therapeutic means to their populations, and which will be at the same time, a source of revenue for the State treasury. Be hold a lot of theories! cry the doctors. Yes, I dream, in my solitude, of things which do not enter into the minds of the physicians; from hence I measure the path, which electro-homeopathy will make in a few years more, by the way that it has made, during the twenty years since it was hardly started. My correspondence, my registers allow me to state, that my discovery is called to regenerate the people, to save, to the budget of the State, the Province, the Commune, the millions now expended in the relief of public suffering, and to increase the receipt of the treasury by the new duty on medicines. I may be deceived, on this point, but I am too well acquainted with the grand reality of electro-homeopathy, and there are too many great personages, who know its reality and its capacity, not to be permitted to believe, that its ultimate destiny is placed in the hands of Governments, to insure its preservation to the word. There I could deposit the formula under the shield of public faith and of persons, who would have only too much interest to perpetuate them and preserve them against every attack.

Until this day arrives, the grand secret must remain unknown and profoundly concealed ; all would be lost, the day it should fall into the hands of those philanthropists, who covet it so uselessly and conceal their spite, when they cry from all sides: Beware of secret remedies!

I have, yet, a categorical word for these brave people: what do you mean by a secret medicine ? According to common sense, it is a medicine, the effects of which are unknown, a medicine which one is afraid to give to publicity, or to the hands of the doctors.

This defined, you call secret, the remedies to which I have given every publicity and, with which, I have supplied every doctor? Remedies, which, for twenty years, I have sent to doctors, chemists, scientific men and the most eminent men in all the countries of the world? Remedies, again, of which the effects, the mode of application, the vegetable and non-poisonous nature are perfectly proved ? Should I not have declared it, every chemist can he not decompose and analyse it? Chemistry, which discovers a grain of poison in the decomposed intestines of a buried dead body ; chemistry which detects the least adulterations, (and even a ten millionth part of a gram of matter does not escape its powerful means of research) could it not detect what there is in my bottles, or in a kilogramme of my granules? It could, with one stroke, tear aside the mysterious veil and annihilate that, which many very serious doctors have called: quackery. Thus it is not logical to reject me, in the name of science; science, on the contrary demonstrates that you have recourse to a ridiculous pretext and one unworthy of serious men.

What interests you is not its nature and effects; it is the material process. I understand that it suits you better. But, then, how many secrets are there not in your official medicine? Is it not from the class of doctors and pharmacists that issue the great part of the secrets which encumber the fly-leaves of the press, the advertisement corners of all towns, the windows of all the pharmacies? Well, the inventors of all these remedies, certainly infallible to cure over loaded purses, have they placed their secret upon the label? What! here you are contented with a name and some details for use, and, especially, that wants no explanation : not to be deceived by the numerous counterfeits. Now why should I, who, according to you, have discovered nothing, and only play the part of a mountebank or ceairvoyant[1], submit to you my process? So much noise for nothing, for an empty secret; this is a new contradiction on your part, or, better still, it is a new proof that this nothing is a great reality which preoccupies you, even to vexation. Without speaking of patented specifies, so much the fashion of our time, of which the inventors preserve the secret, there

1. a person who deceives others, as according to his critics.

are manipulations, in existing preparations, which remain secret to the doctor. The doctor does not require to know the different processes that bark undergoes to furnish sulphate of Quinine; he ought to know that it is the sulphate, and the effect it produces. This is all that he requires; this is also all that I state about my remedies. Every thing else, I repeat, will remain concealed till the day, which myself, or some one after me, shall place it security, in hands which command prisons, to prevent fraud and dishonest trade.

To many readers, mine is certainly a broken language, but there are those who understand my English; those are they, who sigh after my secret; all those, who have taken so much trouble to extort it from me, even sending so many worthy fellows to the neighbourhood of my retreat, to frighten me; all 'those who, to better rove the efficacy of electro homeopathy and the philanthropy of the Count, have demanded a German silver coin for a granule and 800 francs for a litre of electricity, whereas, elsewhere, doctors who were modest, did not take more than 10 francs for an ounce of my fluids ; as for the globules, they settled the affair in such a way as to increase the effect and, especially, the price.

All this was endurable, whilst it was a question of making known the remedies, and, above all, getting them appreciated, when there was no charge, as I sent them gratis ; but now that I sell them, the German silver coin represents 1350 times the cost price at Bologna, and the competition of the inventor has frustrated the projects of the philanthropists throughout the world.

There only remained one attempt to this band.

They said: since the Count guards his person and his formula in his castle, from which we cannot hope to draw them: since he does not, even, allow us to think a little of our purse and our future at the eve of a cataclysm[1] which threatens

1. scientific basis for some old legends.

our position, acquired at the price of study and effort, we will overthrow his grand project.

We must present ourselves as his propagandists; at first we will push the propaganda and gain money; then, after the monopoly will remain to us, or we will overturn the whole. Thus, we shall have done a good thing, in ridding the world of that which the visionary of the Rocchetta called our end, finial to make an end of him, we must distribute good and bad remedies, especially the bad !

Here, adulteration is easy and, when it will be seen and heard that, for one successful case there are so many failures and which, even, show some danger, the sure effects of electro-homeopathy become uncertain ; then some colics caused here and there will put all the world on its guard. Then, the miracles of Bologna and Rome will soon be a matter of legend or mythology; finally, the curable diseases will again become incurable, as it ought to be here below, where it would be difficult to know what to do with the numerous population which would accumulate in the old continent ; it would happen as Malthus has stated.

Finally, the inventor dead, the medicine destroyed, the world will say no more about it.

Behold again more hallucinations ! will exclaim more than one of my readers.

See, however, history that will be written; the documents exist, which I hold, which cannot be easily destroyed, should I, even, be compelled to engrave them on flint.

For the present, I quit history, as I have only one task, that is to insure the world a perfect knowledge of electro-homeopathy, and the purity of the remedies. Adulteration is impossible at Bologna; drawn from the source, it is not exacting too much. So, by very simple means, I think I have baffled even the last scheme, that of all the most dreadful, viz.

adulteration. Have I finished with intrigues[1]? I do not know; but, if after all that I have done, the men, who preside over the destinies of the world, or the societies, accustomed to regard human life as being at their mercy and human suffering as something to be speculated on, so as to make a living out of sickness and death: if, I say, men should find the means of destroying this benefit, which heaven has sent into the world : it would be the occasion to exclaim : men were not worthy of it!

I have faith that ruin will not come ; the remedies that I have discovered will remain ; the attacks and plots of the wicked cannot destroy the truth.

Electro-homeopathy is the truth of medicine. The truth is medicine, after twenty-five centuries of mistakes and errors, is an event -an event which contains the health of generations present and to come, an event which is the integral element of the grand discoveries of the century and of the new order of things, which these discoveries have produced on the face of the globe.

---

1. that cause a reaction in me (referring to the false propagation of his imitators).

Electro-Homeopathy
Medical Part

Observation made by one's self.
The notice of observations of others,
The induction drawn from similars,
Here is the tripod of medicine.

1

What is Electro-Homeopathy?

Electro-homeopathy is homeopathy raised to the perfection of certain and radical medicine by the discovery of new therapeutic agents (which I call electroides), acting on the blood, and giving power to the organism to disengage itself from the morbid principles which change it.

This materia medica has been discovered, like homeopathy, of which it is the crowning point, by experiment; it rests entirely on experimental data; it is therefore true. Like the truth it is also simple. Its effects are explained by principles equally simple.

The body of man is impregnated with certain impurities or principles which some call herpethic, others scrofulous, and which Hahnemann called psoric[1].

---

1. Hahnemann's "Psoric" constitution corresponds to the "carbonic" constitution of Grauvogel. The "syphilitic" constitution to the "Oxygenoid" constitution of Grauvogel. The "Sycotic" constitution to the "Hydrogenoid" constitution of Grauvogel. Count Mattei also came to similar conclusion as regards the essence of the being essentially constitutional (dyscrasia), and the connection between the external phenomenon thereof (Symptoms).

   Below is a graphical presentation of the humors :

Hahnemann	Van Grauvogel	Count Mattei	Dhanwantarti
Syphilis	Oxygenoid	Sanguine	Pitta (Bile)
Sycosis	Hydrogenoid	Lymphatic	Vayu (Wind)
Psora	Carbonitrogenoid	Mixed	Kapha (Phlegm)

These principles vitiate the organization and predispose it to numerous diseases. But there exist, to expel them, remedies which I name antiscrofulous.

This vitiation frequently invades the white vessels, brings on serious changes of the lymph. But there are remedies which I name anti-cancerous.[1] At other times the vitiation gains the sanguine system, produces alteration of the red vessels and diseases the arteries and the veins. There exist remedies that I name anti-vascular, anti angiotic:[2]

With the help of these three kinds of remedies nearly all these maladies can be successfully treated, some other remedies are included in this materia medica[3]:

The Pectorals which have an elective action on the bronchial tubes. The Febrifuges which cure fevers and changes in the liver and spleen. The Vermifuges which destroy intestinal Worms, from the thread worm to the tape worm and tricocephalus. The Antiveneríos which cures syphilis, in all its forms, and perhaps prevents it.

Important remark; In general thesis, there are only two primitive causes of disease (and two classes of remedies) namely: the vitiation of the blood and the vitiation of the lymph. But it ought to be remarked: 1st. That the lymph and the blood are two joint agents in the functions of the organism; the vitiation of one entrains, sooner or later, that of the other ; hence, the mixed diseases which must be attacked by the two classes of remedies alternately: 2nd. The antiscrofulous exert a general action on the lymphatic system as the antiangioitics act on the sanguine. Then it happens that when

1. It will be seen hereafter that the sphere of action of each remedy extends far beyond that which its name literally seems to indicate.

2. From the Greek (angeion) vessel.

3. Electrohomeopathic Medicine by C C Mattei (Originals).

the diseases are fixed and developed to a certain degree, the joint action is, or may be slow to arrest the rapid progress of the complaint.

This is why I have been led to seek specific remedies such as the anticancerous, antivenereal, febrifuges, etc.

These remedies, for me, are only antiscrofulous or antiangiotics, having a more determined, more immediate action either on the lymph or the blood.

This results from experiment, for the antiscrofulous, for example, is a so antivenereal and is sufficient to attack syphilis as long as the disease is only 'developed or arrived to a certain stage. The same is to be said of other specific remedies. The febrifuge combats especially fever; that is to say it restores the normal circulation; but the antiangioitics, acting on disturbances of the blood, also bring back the sanguine tide to its regular rate and thus prevent feverish symptoms, etc.

3. There are also liquids, which powerfully aid the internal treatment and, in many cases, are all that it is required. These fluids have an instantaneous action, similar to that exercised by electricity on the living organism, even in some rare cases producing a shock, I have named them, more particularly, electric fluids or simply electricities.

All these remedies are comprised under the law of similars, in the sense that, given in large doses, they reveal the symptoms of the maladies of which, in proper doses, they eradicate even the cause. But experience does not authorize me to state that they produce morbid symptoms, in a healthy subject, who has no predisposition to or no germ of disease. In this, electro-homeopathy has not hitherto confirmed, in all its generality, the law of Hahnemann.

All these remedies are extracted from non-poisonous plants, as is proved by experiment and analysis.

In ordinary treatment, one globule, daily, is given to a man; this dose is sufficient to cure. But if a hundred, a thousand or a whole bottle of 10,000 granules, are given to a dog, no effect will be observed. A man, in like manner can take, without effect, a certain quantity of granules, providing that the remedy is not appropriate to the disease, which he has, and for which he takes another specific. In this last case, he will perceive unpleasant symptoms, but no danger.

4. It follows, from the preceding, that, the greater the severity of the disease, the smaller should be the dose. This is, moreover, a constant rule, drawn from experience. Thus, an intermittent fever is cured with a grain, in a glass of water, daily ; a malignant fever requires the second or third dilution.

But, aside from the case of certain convulsive diseases, the more dilute the remedy, the more often it must be taken.

So, for the intermittent, it is fit to administer the glass of water, containing the granule, in eight or ten times during the day; whereas, for the malignant, it will be proper to give the granule at the second or third dilution, for several times, a teaspoonful every five minutes, if it is possible.

It is, frequently, proper to give several remedies to the patient; they must not be mixed, nor given at the same time, but alternated by giving, one part of the day, one; the other part of the day, the other.

Tubercles of the lungs, for instance, require the use of anti-cancerous and pectorals ; if there is a spitting of blood, a third remedy is added, chosen from the anti-angioitics. A third of the day ought, then, to be devoted to each of these remedies.

The rule, to select the remedies from this material medica, is as simple as the materia medica itself. Seek the cause of the disease, whatever may be the form, cause which, most often, must be scrofulous, cancerous, or angioitic; and, to this cause, oppose the proper specific.

Thus, for paralysis, the antiangioitics must be employed, if it arises from a defect of the circulation; if it proceeds from the psora or scrofulous principle, the antiscrofuloso is indicated.

In like manner, for the electricities which hasten the internal treatment, those must be chosen which agree with the cause of the disease. If the cause is in the circulation, apply the electricity antiangioitic; the red and the yellow are preferable, if the cause is scrofulous. We shall give, hereafter, more detailed rules for the selection and employment of the remedies.

5. The homeopaths seek the remedy after the symptoms and forms that the malady assumes, and say : for dropsy such a remedy ; for convulsions, such another remedy. This is not the method of electro-homeopathy; for, the same forms of disease may arise from various causes. Thus, convulsions occasioned by worms, could not be treated by a remedy which rectifies the circulation, and vice versa.

Every dropsy could not be cured by one and the same remedy ; that, which cures dropsy of the belly, would not be suitable to dropsy of the heart or of the ovaries. But, in each of these cases, the remedy must be used, which has an elective action on the viscera become the seat of the effusion.

The action which each remedy, applied to the exterior, exercises on the economy, is the same with a degree of difference, as the action of the same remedy, taken internally; a congestion of the liver, for example, will be more quickly subdued, if an external treatment is added to the internal, either by compression or medicated ointment of the same remedy, as given internally, and in doses which will be indicated in this work.

For the same reason, a diminished blood vessel or an aneurism[1], will be more promptly relieved, if compresses or ointments are applied to the affected part, during the internal treatment.

The grave scrofulous or syphilitic maladies, which do not yield to their special remedy, are treated with the anticancerous.

When no effect is obtained, from a remedy, or the effect is slow in showing itself, one of three things is certain; either that the diagnosis is erroneous and the remedy consequently badly selected, or the dose is wrong, or decomposition is so far advanced that it is humanly impossible to succeed.

The effect of the remedy cannot fail, on condition that they are properly given and according to the rules, which we indicate here and which we shall develop further on. With the help of this book, every one can, with a little reflection and observation, be come his own physician and administer this materia medica with success.

---

* tumor-shaped vascular formation located on the tract of an artery or veins.

2

Names of the Electro-Homeopathic Remedies

6. These remedies are now 24 in number ; 19 for internal use, 5 for external. These last are called: electric fluids or simply electroides.

This number has varied, and may yet be increased, as all the remedies have not been discovered at the same time, and there are, at this moment, some, undergoing experiment[1].

List of remedies.

The internal remedies are:

Antiscrofoloso	Antiscrofulous
Antiscrofoloso nuovo or 2°	new or 2d[2].
Antiscrofoloso doppio	double.
Antiscrofoloso 5	5th.

1. There are, at the general dispensary at Bologna: antiscrofuloso 6, anticanceroso 6, pettorale 1, angioilico 3, anticanceroso 10.
2. The new Febrifuge or 2d. although included in the list of internal remedies, is only employed, ordinarily, in compresses or lotions or ointments over the hypochondria's; given in the interior, at the second glass, it has subdued typhus and very serious cases of fever.

Anticanceroso	Anticancerous.
Anticanceroso nuovo or 2°	new or 2d.
Anticanceroso doppio	double.
Anticanceroso 4°	4th.
Anticanceroso 5°	5th.
Antiangioitico	Antangiotic.
Antiangioitico nuovo or 2°	new or 2d.
Pettorale	Pectoral.
Pettorale 2	Pectoral 2d.
Pettorale 3°	Pectoral 3d.
Febrifugo	Febrifuge.
Febrifugo 2°	new or 2d.
Vermifugo	Vermifuge
Vermifugo nuovo	new or 2d
Antivenereo	**Antivenereal**

The external remedies or electricities are:

Red Electricity	Positive.
Yellow Electricty	Negative.
White Electricity	In some way neutral, always beneficial.
Blue or angioitic Electricity.	
Green Electricity	Negative.

Important Remarks:

7. I. *Among the internal remedies, there are three, namely :* antiscrofaloso, anticanceroso, antiangiotico which fill the part of chief remedies ; they are, especially, the main remedies, in

the great majority of diseases, of which the source, as we have so often repeated, is scrofulous, cancerous, or angioitic[1].

Amongst the others, the homonymes[2] are indicated, in peculiar cases, and some have elective action, as will be seen (remark 2.)

The antivenereal acts upon syphilis, in all its forms and all its consequences.

The febrrifuges are specifics against all sorts of fevers, all periodical maladies, and all affections of the liver and spleen.

The pectorals are adapted to affections of the respiratory system.

The vermifuges are employed against every species of intestinal worms.

II. Elective action of certain remedies.

Pectoral 1st acts, in an elective manner, on the bronchial tubes, Pectoral 2nd on the cavities of the lungs, Pectoral 3rd in catarrh.

Anticanceroso 1st acts, in the same way, on spasms of the womb and difficult labors.

Anticanceroso nuovo, against dropsy.

Anticanceroso 4th against decay of the bones.

Antiscrofoloso 1st has an elective action on the stone, calculus and gravel.

Antiscrofoloso nuovo for non-cancerous wounds.

---

1. The antiscrofulous applies to vitiation of the lymph ; the anticancerous to these when they are already far advanced and serious, as in tubercles,cancer etc., the antiangiotics to disorders of the sanguine circulation.
2. a word that is said or spelled the same way as another word but has a different meaning.

Antiscrofoloso 5th in spinal affections.

III. It is always necessary to commence the treatment, by the first remedies, in their series; save to have recourse, afterwards, to their homonymes, when experience shall have shown that the first are not sufficient. After this, it is seen that, with the exception of some cases, every treatment ought to commence with one of the seven following remedies; Antiscrofoloso, Anticanceroso, Antiangioltico, Antivenerio, Febrifugo, Vermifugo, Pettorale.

It is understood that the remedy named and marked, without number or adjective, is the first ; so antiscrofoloso is the same as anticrofoloso 1st ; antiangiotico is identical with antiangioitico 1st. This remark applies, equally, to the nomenclature employed in the books and labels, placed on the bottles containing the remedies.

IV. It must not be forgotten, that the mode of action of the remedies is the same externally as internally, and that, consequently, the cure is hastened by this joint means.

The remedies act rapidly, even instantaneously ; this allows of trials being rapidly made, so as to determine the selection of the remedy.

But it should be noted that, according to the different constitutions and the complication of diseases the sensible and clearly pronounced effects may be, more or less, slow in showing themselves.

V. Finally the blood and the lymph, although circulating in to systems of vessels perfectly distinct, have their common origin in the laboratory of digestion, which furnishes incessantly the materials constituting the pieces of the organization for the maintenance of life.

It results that the diseases of the lymph encroachment upon the blood and vice versa; hence the necessity to have recourse to two or more alternated remedies to insure the cure.

External remedies, or

8. I have, already, sufficiently explained the meaning attached to the words: electric remedies, electricities. Certain physicians, who practice science and not medicine, find, in these words, a sort of scientific profanation; for myself, who never make any question of names, I find sufficient analogy between my remedies and the mode of action of electricity on the organism. These worthy doctors know, without doubt, that the electric current has an instantaneous action ; that the action of the positive pole, is not the same as the negative; that the voltaic wire applied on the extremity of a nerve, excites it directly through its whole length, and by reflection or derivation, the excitement extends throughout the whole of the organism. The doctors, who know all this, have invented words to designate the effects; they have said that the nervous system is found in an electronic state, which state the voltaic current has the power of modifying, so as to render it catelectrotonic or anelectrotonic[1], according to the pole that is considered.

I, also, have sought for words to designate new phenomena, unknown before my time, mysterious even to myself, who discovered them. When I saw that my fluids acted with a rapidity comparable to that of electricity ; when I saw them, in some cases, produce the shock ; when I have remarked that,

---

1. If the polarizing current be opened, so as to stop its passage through the nerve, and remove the anelectrotonic and the catelectrotonic states, a kind of rebound occurs in the condition of both the altered regions, and the part which has just ceased to be catelectrotonic, and was, therefore, over-irritable, becomes, by a kind of negative modification, very much lowered in its irritability; while, on the other hand, the anelectrotonic part, by a positive rebound, becomes more excitable than in its normal state. (source: *A Manual of Physiology* by Gerald F. Yeo, P. Blakiston, Son & Co., 1889)

in touching the great sympathetic at the side of the 7th cervical vertebra, all the pneumo-gastric system was agitated; when I obtains the same effect by placing some granules of antiscrofoloso dry on the tongue; finally, when I observed that one of the liquids in creased the tetanic contractions, whereas another removed them instantly; when I have seen all this, that I describe, and more still. I said: this is positive, negative and neutral electricity, etc.

I abide, by these words, and I do not yet renounce the idea that there is something in it, which may be called electroide or simply electricity, or, it may well be said, that, at the contact of these fluids with the surface of the organism, an electro-motive force, comparable to that which gives issue to the current in galvanic piles, develops itself. What now! have not living bodies their electric currents? And Galvani has he not proved animal electricity, which furnished to the celebrated Mateucci apparatus[1] similar to ordinary electric piles? And, then, is electricity, at this day, so well known, that it must be believed that it is completely and entirely confined to cabinets and Leyden jars? Finally, let it be, that my electricities are found, really innate, in the plants from which they are extracted; let it be, that they are developed by the contact of the juice of these plants with the skin; I choose to call these extra ordinary remedies, these very powerful principles: vegetable electricities.

9. Not wishing to tell all my secrets, obliged however, to state all that is necessary to distinguish the effects, and, above all, to avoid any mistake on the part of the practitioner. I had the electric liquids colored red, straw color, green, blue, etc. I perceived that this expedient rather tended to commercial adulteration ; I no longer color them, but send them out all

1. an instrument designed by Carlo Matteucci proving that electromagnetic induction occurs at large distances and with no ferromagnetic materials.

colorless, or nearly so, only marking on the labels: red, yellow, green, blue, and white electricity; names which I retain, equally, in the nomenclature of the new science.

10. The electricities are only applied, externally, in the manner which will be indicated hereafter ; they are frequently all that is required, when the complaint is external, without any internal lesion or organic alteration. This is the case, with a number of pains; in these cases, it would be wrong to consider them as simple palliatives. In general, the electricities, properly used, lend a powerful support to the treatment and cure, which, in the main, require internal remedies.

3

General Information about the Electro-Homeopathic Remedies

11. All these remedies are extracted from non-poisonous plants, having electric properties in the sense above declared.

They produce a gentle and instantaneous action, but generally, gradual, and of such a sort, that the sensible effects are only produced after some time; this period is, some minutes in acute affections, some days in dull chronic and slow moving maladies. In this, again, there is a resemblance between the remedy and the progress of the disease.

The instantaneous action of the remedies can be proved; let a few granules of antiscrofoloso be given, dry, to a person, fainted away, threatened with paralysis, seized with sea-sickness, dysentry, etc.; the complaint will be seen to disappear instantly. It has happened to me, to relieve from a state of intoxication, persons, who did not leave off drinking, merely by putting globules in their wine.

It has also happened to me to see persons faint away, from contact with the red or yellow electricity ; this happens to hysteric, convulsive and angioitic patients; this cannot always be foreseen. But 8 or 10 globules of antiscrofoloso dry have, always, instantly, arrested this effect.

It is the same, at the commencement of cholera, diphtheria, derangement of the stomach, indigestion, etc.

We have traced the differences and the points of contract between electro-homeopathy and homeopathy, properly so called. Hahnemann, the inventor of the law of similars, did not aim to combat the causes of diseases; he stopped short at the visible manifestations, and only destroyed the symptoms.

Electro-homeopathy applies to the cause itself; it destroys, not only, the evil, but the germ of it also, in such a manner, that the cures, here, are real and radical; and, once relieved from his disease, man has no longer to fear either relapses, reflexions, transformations or morbid reappearances.

This superiority of electro-homeopathy depends on the active principle, contained in the medicine, a principle, in my opinion, electric, which it pleased God to allow me to discover, producing a perfect cure.

At Bologna and at Rome, there are persons, whose cure of maladies, pronounced incurable, now. Dates 10, 12 and 15 years; these persons have never ceased, since then, to enjoy perfect health.

Moreover, the purification of the blood, in most, cases, is seen by the elimination of foreign and morbid principles, which are driven out of the frame, by abundant perspirations, by expectorations, by deposits in the urine, sometimes by the eruption of a series of boils or by diarrhoeas presenting no alarming symptoms an d causing no pain.

It is, especially, in the treatment of wounds, aneurisms, tumours, aches and pains, that it is well to have recourse to external remedies; bearing in mind, that under this form, although increasing the action of the internal medicine, they act like the palliatives of allopathy; therefore, it is necessary to increase the quantity, so as to augment the effect; this is exactly the contrary to the internal remedies.

This is what I wish to make certain electro-homeopaths understand, who abide too closely to minute doses. Do not spare the globules when the treatment calls for large doses; baths, lotions, compresses, to subdue an obstinate or rapidly increasing malady, are neither an excessive extravagance of medicines nor a new evolution in the application of remedies requiring a consumption too costly for persons of small means, as wrote the editor of the Review de Geneve at the publication of my new guide book: *Elettromiopatia, scienza nvova*, etc. Castle Monferrato, 1878. (See the Revue Electro homeopatique de Genéve, 1878, n° 5, and the answer, which I addressed to the editors, dated 4th of July 1878, an answer which I have had published, separately, by P. Bertero, Casale Monferrato, and which these gentlemen refused to insert in the Revue de-Geneve.

4

Sphere of Action of the Remedies in Globules

14. Antiscrofoloso. The antiscrofulous, especially the 1st and the 5th, are the most remarkable, for their power and the extent of their action.

The antiscrofulous tend to annihilate the psoric, herpetic, or scrofulous principles, with which the frame, as has been stated, is more or less impregnated. The principles, naturally, never diminish, and, accumulating without cessation, finish by producing grave infirmities or premature old age. The action of the antiscrofulous, sufficiently prolonged, frees the system from these. This is why these remedies cure ninety out of a hundred diseases; this is, moreover, the result of experience, whence it may be concluded that the greater number of complaints arise from scrofula, which is, in my opinion, hereditary leprosy or syphilis.

It is, for the same reason, that the antiscrofulous prevent disease. The other remedies cut short the disease, at the onset, but they do not prevent it; at least, as far as I know, up to this time ; whereas, the antiscrofulous, is purifying the psoric constitution, prevents the evil from happening.

The antiscrofulous are, therefore, the only remedies that can be taken, preventively, to ward off disease, to strengthen the health by good digestion and calm and restoring sleep, to fortify it against liability to chills, inflammations and a multitude of petty infirmities, which are often the germ of more series complaints.

Entire families, even populations, could protect themselves from many diseases and be regenerated by the daily use of the antiscrofulous, mixed with the food or the water at table.

Some years since, a German prince engaged me to prepare a sanitary project or regulation to revivify the blood of his subjects, by means of electro-homeopathy. But he thought it was necessary to have an understanding with a medical celebrity, who, after having written to me respecting it, with much zeal and enthusiasm, retired at last in a silence, from which, neither the prince nor the people, could make him come forward.

15. Anticancerosi. These remedies display their specific action in all scrofulous complaints, arrived at the most serious sta e, such as : scirrhus, tumours, etc., and which, for his reason, have shown themselves rebellious to the action of antiscrofulous.

The cure of scirrhus and cancer is certain, as long as the essential organs of life have not been, too profoundly, attacked, or the prostration of strength, the evasion of disease and the rapidity of its progress, have not arrived to the point, where there is not left time, necessary for the remedy to purify the blood.

This is what happens, especially, when the fever of absorption has set in. In these extreme cases, the certainty of cure is lost, but not the certainty of soothing, diminishing , relieving the pains and of retarding the hour of death. But it is said:

Principiis obsta, ser medicine paratur

Quum mala per longas invaluere morus[1].

Which is to say that the disease must be subdued at its commencement, and not to wait until the patient is dead or reduced to the impossibility of being cured.

This is the contrary to what is generally done; they wait until the disease is well defined, till the tumour is very large; then they cut it out or give opium to prepare, not medicine, but death. It is certainly this, which with Doctor Peter, professor of internal pathology at the University of Paris, reproaches physicians, exclaiming: This is a crime.

The first effect of the anticancerous is, frequently, the appearance of aggravating the disease ; the reason is in the work itself of the remedy, which stirs up the depth of the frame, to expel the cancerous principles and, in some way to separate the living particles from those which are already in a state of decomposed elements.

Sometimes, also, the good effect appears to stop, during the time necessary for the remedy to penetrate and saturate, so to say, the organism. But the point of saturation arrived at, the cure commences and progresses more and more rapidly. The treatment of these diseases may last months, sometimes years, more or less time according to the mischief to subdue. Particular difficulties may be the disease, may remain stationary ; even partial relapses may happen, but this must not discourage you ; perseverance will end by prevailing, and will prevail as much as is humanly possible, as the remedies never fail.

Once commenced, the cure of cancer must never be interrupted; it would be exposed to irreparable relapses. I say this from knowledged of the cause; let attention be paid to it.

---

1. stop it at the beginnings: it is too late to employ medicine when the illness has gain strength. - Ovid, Remedia Amoris, XCI.

The anticancerous which gives the best result in the treatment of cancer are: anticanceroso 1, anticanceroso 4, and anticanceroso 5[1].

16. Antiangioitico.-These remedies are the regulators and purifiers of the blood; they act on the whole system of circulation, principally on the heart and its diseases.

From the reason that vitiations of the blood cause corresponding vitiations of the lymph and vice versa, it is frequently necessary, in practice, to alternate the antiangioitics with the antiscrofulous, or with the anticancerous, or with the specific remedies. Thus, when in certain changes in the sanguine system, such as vericose veins, hypertrophy of the heart, etc., congestion of the liver, is present as the same time, for which the febrifuges are specific, they must be alternated, either externally or internally, with the antiangioitics.

When the electricities otherwise indicated produce no effect, the existence of a serious change in the blood or circulation may be suspected.

In this case, compresses, lotions or baths of antiangioitics may be advantageously substituted for the electricities.

17. Antivenereo- is the specific for the cure of syphilis and all its results, even the most serious and the most remote.

It is employed, consequently, in the treatment of hereditary syphilis and the numerous maladies resulting from it. Many complaints, many scrofulous and cancerous affections have their secret source in a syphilitic heritage. In all these cases antiscrofoloso also acts as an antisyphilitic, but it will be advantageous to alternate the anticenereo with the antiscrofulous and the anticancerous.

---

1. Recently, I have obtained very good results, in the treatment of the cancer, by giving canceroso 10, a remedy newly discovered.

Cases of syphilis, properly so called, which do not yield to the antivenereo should be treated by the anticancerous.

18. Febrifugo-The febrifuges are appropriate to intermittent, pernicious and inflammatory fevers and, in general, to every sort of fever, even those simply symptomatic.

These remedies are much more certain (and especially without danger) than sulphate of quinine and aconite.

Persons dying from typhoid fever, arrived at the gates of death, already given up as dead, have been brought back to life and cured by small doses of febrifuges, introduced into the mouth already locked, by means of a rag dipped in the remedy or with a teaspoon.

The febrifuges are also specifics against affections of the intermittent type, neuralgia, pains, etc., and even against maladies of the liver and spleen, with or without accompanying inflammation of the stomach; against congestions, indurations of the viscera, either ancient or recent.

Enormous and obstinate enlargements of the hepatic tissue I have seen dispersed by the febrifuges.

Administered against the fever, at the beginning of an illness which is not determined, they are frequently able to arrest this and when they cannot prevent they certainly mitigate it.

Compresses or lotions prepared with the febrifugo nuova and applied over the region of the spleen give excellent results in every class of infirmity, which ought to be sufficient to demonstrate the importance of this organ, to which the physiologists have not as signed a part. But there is more than one dark spot in classic medicine, on which light will be thrown by the effects of the new remedies. The classic divisions of diseases have no longer a real value in many in stances, as the effects of the antiscrofulous, point out, clearly, the common origin of many complaints apparently the most diverse.

19. Vermifugo-The vermifuges are specifics against all the variety of parasitical diseases: thread worms, tape worms, tricocephalus, etc., and all disorders caused by their presence in the intestines. Occasionally good results have been obtained from these remedies in cases of lumbago and even cancer.

20. Pettorale -The pectorals, as their name indicates, serve in diseases of the chest, the throat, the bronchial tubes and the respiratory organs generally.

They are employed against cough, catarrh, inflammation of the lungs, pleurisy and pulmonary consumption.

We have already noted the elective action shown by the pectorals 1, 2, 3; (see chapter II, note 11.)

5

General Remarks on the Electric Liquids, Their Mode of Application

21. These liquids are also extracted from non-poisonous plants, having powerful properties or principles which resemble electric force, in a word, they are a class of electroides.

These liquids, unchangeable as all my remedies, are five in number, viz:

Red electricity-having positive action.

Yellow-having negative action.

White-of which the action in some way mixed or neutral, is always beneficial.

Blue or angioitic-positive, but especially adapted to angioitic persons, who cannot support the red or the yellow.

Green-negative, especially adapted to cancerous wounds.

The electricities are, generally, employed externally or subcutaneously. The various species of electricities produce actions differing in nature, but all of equal power; a power, which is, more or less; felt by different temperaments and according to their degree of vitiation.

This action is rapid, sometimes instantaneous; in rarer cases it produces a shock, as electricity properly so called in twenty years it has happened to me to see this singular phenomenon 8 or 10 times, but it must also be noted that, generally, you have to do with persons who have not the habit of notice.

The most remarkable and most precious effect of the vegetable electricities are to sooth and, frequently, to remove pain completely without disturbing the constitution.

22. Certain diseases, when they do not proceed from a too far advanced vitiation of the lymph or the blood, are rapidly and often instantly cured by the application of electricity only. This is how I have cured partial tetanus by applying yellow electricity to the back of the head in the same way, by the electricities alone properly used, I have cured by hundreds, cases of amaurosis, chronic cephalalgia, rheumatism, sciatica, articular pains, and stammering from the birth in a person aged 45 years.

Science has recognized the reciprocal influence of the blood on the nerves, and the nerves on the blood.

The cures by the electricities alone (which act on the nerves) demonstrate surely the influence of the nerves on the blood. The disappearance of certain nervous affections by single remedies which purify the blood, point out, on the other hand, the influence of the blood on the nerves.

'I have not yet met with a single contradiction be tween the truths of the new art, and the truth, really such, recognized by science.'

The vegetable electricities alone cannot cure constitutional maladies; for these, internal treatment is indispensable.

But even in these cases, these liquids, joined to the internal treatment, are a powerful assistance to hasten the cure and to shorten the period of convalescence.

Health, as we have before said, is the result of a certain equilibrium between all the powers of, the organism; there was some truth in the system of Brown (which has been so much abused) reducing all diseases to sthenia asthenia. We are ill by excess, or default; health is the just medium. This is why I have found so much a vantage in alternating the positive red Electricity with the negative yellow, especially in convalescence. The organic functions are thus powerfully excited in the infirm parts, by increasing at first t e vital power, then withdrawing the excess of this power and bringing back the organism, in this way, to a state of equilibrium.

The suppression or at least the mitigation of pain is, already, an estimable benefit which the vegetable electricities bring to a multitude of diseases, particularly in the ulcerations of cancer, in sores and wounds of every description. If I had only found this mean of relieving suffering, should I not have had reason to thank God and to continue to proclaim it to the world ?

It is particularly in the treatment of scrofulous maladies that the use of the electricities supports the action of the internal remedies and produces the best results.

23. Mode of application of the electricities. The electricities are used either as compresses, by Soaking a piece of linen in a few drops which are at once applied to the art indicated, or as a cupping glass by reversing the bottle holding the liquid and applying its mouth to the place where it is required to act.

The Yellow electricity is only applied as cupping.

The Red:	positive	Employed either as compress or as cupping.
The White:	positive[1]	
The Blue:	positive	
The Green:	negative	

Points of application:

The points of application of the electricities are, generally, indicated by the seat of the pain or injury (contusions, wounds, sores, etc.).

In all cases, take care to touch the parts where the nerves are nearest to the skin or the pain; according to this rule the plate, at the end of the volume, is drawn and which we supposed to be now before us.

To act on the whole body: touch the occiput, the great sympathetic, along the spine each side where the nerves issue, and under the arch of the foot.

To act on the right side of the head: apply to the right temple, forehead, upper and under orbital, and root of the nose.

For the left side: choose the homologous points of this side.

For the tongue: the great and especially the small hypoglossids.

For the eyes: to the occiput, to the great sympathetic, to the sub and super orbital.

For the nose: to the root of the nose between the eyes, to the occiput, to the super and sub orbital.

For the ears: to the three little muscles behind the ear, but especially to the bottom of the ear.

For this open the mouth and apply compresses of red or white electricity to the place where the ear joins the jawbone. The positive electricities can, also be used as gargles, but never the yellow or green.

1. Cesare Mattei however throughout maintained that W.E. is neutral, strange that here W.E. is marked as positive, quite contradictory.

For the arm: see the marks on the plate.

For the leg: see the plate, and also touch the sacred nerves, at the sides of the spine at the height of about 8 inches counting from the bottom, and under the arch of the foot.

To act on the bladder, the womb, etc.: apply to the sacred nerves, the perineum, the pubis and the great sympathetic nerve.

The seat of pain generally indicates the point that ought to be touched, little custom will teach the rest; 1 The duration of the application: as cupping it varies from 3 to 20 seconds. The applications of 7, 10 and 15 seconds are usually the most efficacious; short and frequent act the best. The compresses are left until dry and renewed more or less often, according to the effect. The compress is prepared by moistening about a square inch of clean linen, but the dimensions, and the quantity of liquid, vary according to the extent of the sore or the surface of the application.

24. When it is a question of pain, commence always with the electricity ; if the pain returns, join the internal treatment to the electric applications.

Usually, it is the red that is first applied; for most times, man is ill for want of vitality, he is negative. The red is alternated with the yellow to bring back the neutral state, health. These alternations are especially efficacious in convalescence.

When pain is to be removed, always wait to see the effect of the red before going on to the yellow.

But to remove a humour, to act simply on the organism the applications of the red and the yellow follow each other immediately.

When neither the red nor the yellow produce any effect, make compresses (specially for the head) with the white which always does good. If neither of these three not, there exists a vitiation of the blood or the lymph, for without this, one of the three would certainly have produced a result.

The blue electricity is reserved for the sanguine temperaments, which ought to be studied in advance, for the purely sanguine temperaments, when invalid, may feel; from the use of the red and the yellow, disturbances which, although only temporary, ought to be avoided. For these persons all the electricities are replaced by the angiotic electricity. The greatest utility of this is seen in wounds; good compresses remove pain, stops the bleeding, and cicatrises[1] even the wounded arteries. For the wounds very strong compresses of this electricity are necessary[2]. The green electricity, in compresses, is particularly suitable for calming the pain of ulcerated cancer; it is used pure, or mixed with water, according to the necessity and the effect. It is applicable to all sorts of wounds, especially for articular pains which on the onset, it subdues in every case; it is necessary to regulate the quantity according to the constitution.

---

1. scars left by the formation of new connective tissue over a healing sore or wound.

2. In consequence of a wound in the bronchial artery. which the doctor did not know how to dress, after 18 days of haemorrhage the patient was dying. Good compress of the blue electricity stopped the blood, and even cicatrised the artery: the man was saved. This is a fact which formerly would have appeared impossible.

6

Results of Experience

25. Prostration of strength is increased by the application of the yellow electricity; on the contrary, the red re-establishes the strength, sometimes instantly, at the first touch. In a case of partial tetanus caused by a wound, the yellow electricity, applied to the occiput, the great sympathetic and injured part, immediately relaxed the tension of the nerves whereas the red had increased it.

It is on similar phenomena, constantly observed, that I base the denominations of positive and negative vegetable electricity.

In acute diseases, these electricities, properly managed, render the greatest service. Thus, in violent erysipelas of the face, applications of red electricity to the occiput, great sympathetic, forehead, and super and sub orbital nerves, aided by scrofoloso 1 internally, cause the pain, inflammation, fever and other symptoms to disappear.

In the same manner, in stitch in the side, inflammation of the breasts, pleurisy, electricity to the sympathetic and the solar plexus with scrofoloso 1 and pettorale 1, internally, overthrow the fever, oppression, pain and all the most serious symptoms.

In very acute sciatica, if electricity, applied to the sciatic and sacral nerves, does not succeed, employ lotions with the anticancerous 5 and antiangioitic 2 alternately.

In apoplexies, it is necessary to pay attention to the cause so as to select the fit electricity, as the electricities, which suit in nervous apoplexy, cannot be employed without danger in sanguine apoplexy.

The beneficial influence of the electricities, as an adjunct to the internal treatment, is seen in a sensible manner; for example, in erysipelas of the face, the eye can follow the decline of the swelling; in opthalmia (cataract), applications to the occiput, to the sympathetic, the root of the nose, the eyes, re-establish the flow of tears; the swelling and inflammation diminish. In wounds, also, the vegetable electricity promotes the flow of humours and the formation of pus.

7

Doses and Method of Administration of the Remedies in Globules

26. I am going to give here general indications as to the doses of the remedies; but absolute rules can not be given, as constitutions vary in finitely; numerous exceptions may occur which must be left to individual observation.

The ordinary dose, for an internal remedy, is fixed at one globule of the first dilution, daily. The second dilution suits better in many cases, especially for women and all persons exceptionally sensitive.

In addition to the grain of the first dilution, in certain cases, from 10 to 20 globules are given dry, either of the same or another remedy; in the last case alternating it with the remedy dissolved in water. I only give the third dilution in extremely violent cases, such as hysteria, epilepsy, typhus, etc.

Dilutions:

The first dilution is obtained by dissolving a globule in a pint glass of drinking water[1]; we also call it the first glass.

---

1. A pint glass is a form of drinkware made to hold either a British (imperial) pint of 20 imperial fluid ounces (568 ml) or an American pint of 16 US fluid ounces.

To make the second dilution, take a teaspoonful of the first, put it into a second pint glass which is to be filled with pure water. This is the second glass. The third is prepared in like manner by taking a teaspoonful of the second glass.

The remedy is taken by teaspoonfuls in such a way as to finish the prescribed quantity in the day.

It must be remembered that the dose ought to be diminished in proportion to the gravity or violence of the disease, and that the more the dose is lessened the more frequently the teaspoonfuls must be administered.

Thus the first dilution would be taken, for an intermittent fever, by exhausting times; for typhus a teaspoonful of the second dilution would be given every 5 or 7 minutes.

27. *External use:*

The granules are used externally in different ways, namely, baths, compresses, lotions, ointments and gargles.

To medicate an ordinary bath (soft water) dissolve a 100, 150, 200 granules in a glass, separately, then add this solution to the bath.

For compresses and gargles, dissolve 20 globules in an ordinary glass of water.

For lotions, dissolve 5 granules in a little water; add a spoonful of oil or lard without salt, and mix thoroughly. Electricities are also used for Baths and Gargles. The proportion is 3 tablespoonsful of electricity for the bath, and 8 to 10 drops for a gargle. The compresses should be renewed three times daily, or oftener according to the effect. We have no need to repeat that the external action of the Granules is the same as the internal.

The doses should be increased in proportion as the disease diminishes, from the reason that the remedy follows the law of similars, or let it be so, acts homeopathically.

But individual perception and habit must do the greater part in regulating the larger or smaller dose required.

Here are rules drawn from experience which it will be useful to read carefully.

I. If the remedy is wrong, it has no effect; if, on the contrary, it produces aggravation, the remedy is found, but the dose must be lessened until no aggravation is produced.

II. The effects of a remedy are not doubtful; they are certain, provided it is directed to a disease included within its sphere of action. Consequently, if after some spoonfuls nothing is observed, or if in spite of the diminution of the close, there is still aggravation, it may be concluded that the remedy is not specific for the malady.

III. The aggravation in such cases is temporary and not dangerous. The patient may feel it in different ways.

But, either by the reduction of the dose or the change of remedy you can always succeed.

These are trials, inevitable preliminary experiments, which a little custom will render easy.

IV. The small doses do not decrease the action of a remedy; they only place it in proportion to the state of the patient.

To infants whilst sucking the remedy is administered to the nurse; for young children the second dilution is employed.

The necessity of taking the remedies in the low dilution and of frequently repeating the spoonfuls in serious conditions, is explained by the fact that the remedies have an instantaneous action which terminates at once; therefore it must be the more frequently repeated to arrive at a satisfactory conclusion.

Experience has shown that the surplus taken is so much lost for the curative effect.

V. The remedy is continued to be taken up to the time of a meal, and even during the repast; the example, before quoted, of a drunken man who, going on drinking, after I had mixed the remedy with his wine, finished by becoming sober, demonstrates that the remedies act the same, even when mixed with the food or drink.

VI. Menstruation is not a reason to discontinue the use of the remedies; on the contrary, it is the most favorable period, as they only act better at this time when the blood acts to expel morbid principles.

Only it is necessary to know that the antiangioitics, in ordinary dose, bring back suppressed menstruation, whereas, in small doses, they are specific against the opposite excess of too great an abundance of menstrual blood, and against general haemorrhage.

VII. The only diet is a healthy and sufficient nourishment; in grave maladies powerful acids, such as vinegar and lemons, must be refrained from.

The remedies are never mixed; compresses and lotions of two different remedies ought to be made successively.

In the same way, when in complicated diseases several remedies are used, they must be given separately and successively, taking care to alternate them.

Seeing that the action of each spoonful of a remedy is of short duration, it is not strictly necessary to reserve an entire part of the day to each of these remedies that are alternated; they can be alternated by following up a spoonful of the first with one of the second, and then recommence by the first and continue with the second, and so on, at the prescribed intervals. The water of the compresses or bath, also for internal use, can be cold, lukewarm, or more or less warm, according to one's taste. It can also be sweetened with sugar, etc.

Here are some rules by means of which any man who knows how to make a diagnosis, that is to say, knows how to distinguish between a lymphatic subject and a sanguine, can suitably administer phase remedies.

VIII. A woman, having a cancer in the breast subject to haemorrhages, sees them increased by having put two granules in her glass, instead of one. The accident disappears as soon as she returns to the prescribed dose; but, anxious to be cured, she again doubles the quantity; the haemorrage recommences and again subsides under the influence of angioitico 2, and cancerous 1, in ordinary doses.

I have seen many similar cases which are very instructive.

For weak and serious patients, it is always prudent to commence by the second dilution, so as to increase them after.

There are cases where feeble doses, the third for example, are absolutely necessary ; such are: organic diseases of the heart, epilepsy, hysteria and convulsive diseases in general.

In other cases, very large doses can be boldly used; 20 or 30 globules dry on the tongue, at the onset of cholera, generally arrest it; the same may be used in asphyxia and other affections.

Finally, there are persons whom it suits better to take eight or ten globules dry, one every hour, in stead of the dilution. These are particular cases depending on differences of constitution and for which is necessary to refer to individual observation. But, in serious diseases, it is of great importance to adhere to the prescribed doses.

8

Of Diagnosis, Principles and Rules for the Selection of the Appropriate Remedy

1 After that which we have so often stated in this book, we will- not further insist upon the experimental principle which ought to guide the-diagnosis and 'lead us to the selection of the specific remedy.

The source of life is in the blood and the lymph; nine times out of ten, the seat of diseases, be the form what it may, is in the vitiation of the lymph; once it is in the vitiation of the blood, or a combined vitiation, from the reciprocal effects of the two constituent elements of the organism.

As there are only these three causes of disease, there can only exist three kinds of ailments; for diagnosis, everything is reduced to this, to know if the patient belongs to one of the three following classes.

1. Lymphatics, by far the most numerous;
2. Angiotics;
3. Combined, which belong to the two proceeding classes by the junction of the vitiation of both, the blood and the lymph, at the same time.

Practically, diagnosis is reduced to ascertain simply if the patient is angiotic or not. If he is, the remedies are antiangiotics, no matter what may be the form of his disease.

The angiotic condition is easily recognized; it is particularly characterized by a florid[1] complexion, tendency to hoemorrhages, congestions, vertigo, palpitations, rapid pulsations in the carotids, haemorrhoids, varicose veins, etc.

If the patient has absolutely none of these symptoms, he is necessarily lymphatic. The antiscrofulous will be his remedy, whatever the disease.

Finally, by the side of some angiotic symptoms one or more, proper to the lymphatics, may be present, such as tumours, enlarged glands, eruptions on the skin, etc. ; it is that the vitiation of the blood co-exist with that of the lymph ; it is a combined disease. The remedies, therefore, are antiscrofulous, and anticancerous combined with antiangiotics.

Most times one will hardly hesitate to choose between the antiscrofulous and the anticancerous.

When the patient has congestion or suppuration of the glands, scrofulous, gangrenous or cancerous wounds, scirrhus, tumours, cancer etc., the main specifics are certainly in the series of anticancerous: other remedies may aid or vary the treatment, but the anticancerous can not be laid aside or suspended.

29. These are the rules that remain fixed for the clearly defined cases. There are those which are not ; when there is a doubt whether the patient is lymphatic, or angiotic, the disease must be treated as combined.

To know the constitution of a patient, it is proper to be acquainted with the previous state of his health, the diseases which he may have had in his infancy, in his youth, and the causes which produced them.

---

1. red-faced person or whose face has turned red with exertion.

Also the health and diseases of the parents may furnish indications, for we all inherit more or less of the constitution of our parents.

It is not difficult to distinguish the affections of the lungs or the disease of the liver; and the afflictions, caused by syphilis, are not easily confounded with the disturbances occasioned by worms. In short, if we meet with cases which embarrass us, it is the same for the physicians, and much more so, as, in their system, diagnosis requires so much skill that it is rare for two or three doctors to pronounce the same opinion in complicated cases, especially if they are consulted separately.

The very great advantage of electro-homeopathy is the power, when there is doubt, to sustain for a period, (which is very short) the treatment by some remedy which, although not the specific, may be the means of finding it; it will be the antiscrofulous 1 and 5 which may generally be tried in these cases.

Hesitation is more frequent in diseases of the liver and spleen and those caused by worms, particularly the tape worm, for nothing is more obscure than these maladies; physicians are deceived nearly as often as the lay. But the electro-homeopathy can, at least, relieve himself from perplexity in these complaints, by administering the vermifugo internally and applying the febrifugo nuovo in compresses to the hypochondria. The effects will soon show the nature oil the disease. The persistance of certain complaints is, sometimes, attached to an obscure hereditary syphilitic taint; when it may be doubtful, alternate antivenereo with the appropriate specific. It is a rule to follow, particularly in certain cancers, scirrhus, doubtful sores; never forgetting however that anticanceroso 1 is also specific against ancient syphilitic virus.

In this case one must be guided by the effects; if the remedies, although well selected and administered, are not successful, it is certain that it is the question of a case properly incurable. There are such, and electro-homeopathy, although relieving them and extending the boundary of the possible, cannot perform the impossible. It works possible miracles by the cure of diseases, even the most cruel, pronounced incurable by allopathy; but on the condition that recource is had to electro-homeopathic remedies before the entire mass of the blood is corrupted, or the essential organs of life seriously deranged. This is the boundary of electro-homeopathy and there also, I think, ends the power of man.

36. Further on follows a catalogue of diseases which have been cured by my remedies, with the indication of all the modes of employing them in similar cases. This variety of means, which the Revue electro-homeopathique of Geneva, year 1878, 11° 5, has condemned being an excessive extravagance of medicines, demonstrates only one thing, namely, that the same complaint cannot always be cured by the remedy; that which has been successful in one case, may not be so, in another, from the very simple reason, that constitutions differ, and the complications of disease are endless. No medication, let it be ever so detailed, can fix an absolute rule for every case; this would be a sort of universal remedy, which can never exist as long as there are organic irregularities in our race.

The treatment of diseases would be very convenient and simple; all that I have written, here and else where, would be almost useless, if the whole affair was reduced to searching, on a synoptical chart[1], the disease and its remedy side by side. No, it is not in this manner that we understand the affair; this is why we have placed, at the side of each disease, not one,

1. Synoptical Chart of Diseases and Corresponding Remedies is given in Principles & Art of Cure in Electrohomeopathy by Debasish Kundu (Originals, New Delhi).

but several means of subduing it. But, we have not said that all these means, and even those which did not yet exist, had been employed in the treatment of patients whose cures are reported in the catalogue. It is astonishing that writers, who had deserved so well of electro-homeopathy, who knew my discoveries by my treatises and my private correspondance, could be so much mistaken as to say in the Rome, that. I gave the credit of the cures, obtained some years ago, the remedies which did not yet exist. The. author of the criticism in 11° 5 of the Revue had well reason to state that: which could care, can still cure; but to cure in all possible cases, it is necessary to be acquainted with the means possible.

And as 1 only preserve silence as regards the formula; I think its my duty to make the people acquainted with all my therapeutic resources, so that it may have the least possible need of doctors either of the old or new school.

9

Easy Experiments for Beginners

31. Amongst those who have seen Electro-homeopathy at work, there are common ignorant people, earned physicians, intelligent and unprejudiced persons belonging to all classes of society.

The ignorant said; it is St. Anthony!

The physicians said; it is nothing!

The persons of good faith said; it is very serious, it is wonderful!

I understand the doctors; I renounce their conversation.

But the intelligent and unprejudiced men have not all seen; the greater number have heard say, have read, or will read electro-homeopathy; they have need to behold, and to behold it, it is sufficient to make a trial.

Here, now, are experiments easy to perform every where.

1. Eight or ten granules of antiscrofulous, placed dry in the mouth of a drunken man, render him sober, arrest a threatening of paralysis or a fainting fit.
2. Two or three granules of the same remedy, on the tongue, restore an interrupted or difficult digestion, give appetite, produce sleep, stop cramp of the stomach, calm the toothache, etc.

3. A few spoonfuls of anticanceroso 1, second dilution, arrest, most frequently in a moment, spasms of the womb; and this same remedy, continued sufficiently long, relieves woman from all the uneasiness felt before, during and after confinement. The same, also, aids delivery in an interrupted labor.
4. Strong compresses of angioitic electricity removes the pain, stop the bleeding of a wound, close and heal it, etc.
5. A few compresses of white electricity remove, instantly neuralgia of the head; a gargle is very often sufficient to carry off the toothache, although of long standing, etc.
6. A healing, continued over a sufficient time with antiscrofoloso 1, and applications of red electricity expels the stone in a sort of gruel, closes ruptures, brings back the fresh color and health in patients of iron-deficiency anemia.
7. With febrifuge 1, internally, and lotions over the hypochondria with the febrifugo nuovo, one removes fevers and all diseases of the liver.

Here are little miracles which the beginners can perform to convince themselves and demonstrate electro-homeopathy; and to acquire, at the same time, confidence and custom to manipulate the remedies, others can also be selected in the list of ailments which follows.

32. It is very generally thought that it is necessary to have confidence, faith, to feel the good effects of the remedies; the allopaths say that, in homeopathy, 'faith is everything. But that is no medicine, of which is to be said: Faith alone is sufficient. Is it faith or confidence that cures the suckling in giving the medicine to the nurse only ? What faith can a man have, dead drunk, a person fainted away, a madman, etc., whose revival to life, however, is not less certain, or prompt? There is no absurdity that has not been said by these men who have eyes and yet see not.

Without doubt, confidence is necessary, not for the effect of the remedy, but to follow out the prescriptions in a serious manner. Faith is especially necessary to beginners, not to add a few grains more in the glass, seeing how small they are; confidence is necessary to persevere the proper time, to avoid the temptation of making a quicker cure with strong doses. Confidence is only necessary at the commencement; after it has been seen, conviction and assurance are acquired.

It is now to recommend every person who begins, not to commence with desperate or extremely difficult cases, which might well be amidst the number of those that are impossible. A check for a beginner, especially in difficult cases, certainly does not overthrow the remedies, but it may discourage the novice and expose him to the jests of those persons who find it always more convenient to ridicule than to conscientiously examine new truths. It does not require a long time to acquire tact and custom, to render oneself acquainted with the remedies; then one can treat difficult cases with success.

Facility and simplicity is not the least prize of this medicine, born and made for the people.

The catalogue of diseases which follows is made so that every man, if he wishes it, may become his own physician; 'medicus esto tibi'[1], according to the proverb of the school of Salerno[2].

Finally, to facilitate this to the people, we borrow, from that excellent little book: The People's Physician, by Doctor Mure[3], a short popular instruction designed to make known the organs contained in the abdomen and the thorax, which will be useful for the practice of electro-homeopathy.

---

1. 'Let each man be his own physician'
2. Schola Medica Salernitana (Italian: Scuola Medica Salernitana) was a late medieval medical school, situated on the Tyrrhenian Sea in the south Italian city of Salerno.
3. Dr. J. B. Mure, author of 'Doctrine del' École de Rio de Janeiro et Pathogénésies Brésiliennes', Paris, 1849.

33. A person of a regular constitution, standing upright, placing the hands, naturally open, on the sides of the belly, the thumbs, directed backwards, towards the vertebral column, the other fingers to the front and opened, the palm of the hands resting on the flanks, the internal edge (the lower in this position) resting on the bones of the hip, the index fingers touching the ribs; we have, in contact with the thumbs, the external edges and the upper extremities of the loins.

The stomach is between the two index fingers, the right index corresponds to the right lobe of the liver and the gall bladder, the left covers the spleen, and extends to the spot where the false ribs cover the left lobe of the liver.

Between the points of the two middle fingers is the transversal colon, that of the right covers the ascending, colon, that of the left the descending colon. The little finger of the right hand rests and the coecum[1], and the left on the iliacs of the colon. Between the ascending transversal and descending colon and the pubis is the mass of the small bowels and their adjuncts.

Behind the pubis, is the bladder which is raised above it when full. Behind the bladder is the rectum and between these, in woman, is the uterus. In a women, the ovaries are under the little fingers, but, during pregnancy, the enlargement of the womb changes all this. The same may be said of over fat persons, swollen or dropsical. This description is only sure for persons of an ordinary constitution.

The organs contained in the chest are more easy to recognize. On each side are the lungs, each enveloped in a serous membrane, called the pleura, like a sort of sack. Between these and a little to the left, is the heart, the point of which beats between the sixth and seventh rib.

---

1. from which the colon originates, and in which the ileum terminates.

Catalogue of Diseases Cured by Electro-Homeopathy

with the indication of all remedies suitable in similar cases

Preliminary and Important Observations

I. We have arranged the diseases in alphabetical order, to facilitate the search, without taking into account the fundamental principle of electro-homeopathy, that: every disease is lymphatic, angiotic or combined. At the side of each disease and its varieties, we have placed the treatment by one or more remedies and their modes of application.

II. It must once more be remembered that: the remedy which has been successful in a case may not in fallibly cure in all possible cases. Hence the necessity of indicating, not only one, but a series of medicines for each disease.

III. It is always understood that to practice electro-homeopathy it is necessary to become thoroughly versed in the preceding principles and rules; after wards, the catalogue may be consulted with advantage and, in it, every one can discern the treatment suitable to each individual case.

IV. With the exception of particular cases, clearly defined, in which individual judgement may recommend some variations, the treatment should always be commenced with the first remedy indicated in the catalogue. When experience (which may last some minutes or days) has proved that the first remedy is not sufficient, recourse must be had to the following ones.

V. The diseases, here reported, have been cured by my remedies; but I report neither the number of cases, nor the different forms, nor the age, name, and rank of persons treated at Bologna, Rome, Rochetta and in foreign countries. All these details can be found in my pamphlet: Un poco di storia sui rimedii Mattei.

VI. For the method of preparing the dilutions, baths, compresses, lotions, gargles, either with the globules or with the vegetable electricities, refer to chapter V for the electricities, and chapter VII for the globules. Finally, for the sake of brevity, we adopt some abridged notations, simple and convenient, and with which the reader should render himself familiar.

Signs and Abbreviations

34. The names of the remedies are indicated by the initial capital letter of their Italian name after omitting the preposition (anti if necessary. Thus one will write:

S for anti-scrofoloso

C for anticanceroso

A for antiangioitico

Ven. for antivenereo

Ver. for vermifugo

F for febrifugo

P for pettorale.

The rank or number of the homonymes is indicated by the arabic cipher placed at the head of the letter as an exponent in algebra; it is not necessary to note the first ones. Thus in this way:

S, S5, S2 denote scrofuloso 1, 5, 2 or nuovo.

A, A2 designate angioitico 1, 2 or nuovo.

In the same way, the anticancerous are denoted as follows:

C, C2 or nuovo, C3 or doppio, C4, C5, etc.

The second and third dilutions will be marked by the indices II, III, placed at the foot of the signs.

The first dilution is not noted, it is understood. Thus,

S signifies scrofoloso first dilution.

S II, S III, signify the remedy at the second and third dilution.

A 2 II signifies angioitico nuovo or 2 at the second dilution.

C 5 III is canceroso 5, taken in the third dilution and so on, for the others.

The signs for the five electricities[1] are:

El, R. Red electricity.

El, J, Yellow electricity.

El, A, Angioitic or blue electricity.

El, V, Green electricity.

El. B, White electricity.

To note that two of the remedies must be alter nated, the sign "—" is used placed between the indication of the remedies, for example;

S "—" A signifies: scrofoloso alternated with an gioitico; S "—" A2 II "—" P II, signifies: scrofoloso, first dilution, alternated with angioitico 2 and pettorale, the two last, both, second dilution.

El. R. "—" El. J. marks the alternation with red and yellow electricity, etc.

Abbreviations:

Compr. compresses

Onct. lotions

Garg. gargles

---

* In Italian Rossa or Rosso, Jiallo or Giallo, Verde and Bianca or Bianco respectively.

For the points of application of the electricities, marked on the figures in the diagram at the end of the book, we frequently use the following abbreviations:

Occ. Occiput.

Simp. Grand sympathetic nerve.

Plex. Sol. Solar plexus.

Sus. orb. Super orbital.

Sous-orb. Sub. orbital.

Hypoc. Hypochondria.

a. b. s. to take frequently, a teaspoonful every 12 or 15 minutes, remembering what is stated chapter VII, -n° 26.

When 20 g. 10 g., etc., are marked, it means 20 or 10 globules, dry, to be taken daily, one every hour or half hour.

In our catalogue the following remedies will be noted only. S. S5. S2. A. A2. C. C2. C4. C5. F. F2. P. P2. or P3. Ver. Ven.

There are other remedies which it is as well to have for particular cases, but these, in addition to the five electricities, are generally sufficient for a domestic medicine chest.

In general, we shall hardly indicate more than the technical name of the diseases, except some cases which require some summary indications; more details would too much increase the size of this manual.

For further information, refer to manuals of pathology, particularly the medeci'n du peuble by Dr. Mure, the fownulaire homeopathique of Frost Lacuzon, and persons who wish for more extended information, the ele'rrmits de medecine pratique by Dr. P. Jousset, Paris 1868. J. B. Bailliére et fils. But we repeat that the simplicity of our new medical science dispenses, in the great majority of cases, with this knowledge and enables every man, who can distinguish a sanguine from a lymphatic constitution, to succeed in his treatment, without troubling himself about learned classifications of diseases, forms and numerous symptoms, in which, the most skilful are frequently embarrassed by the diagnosis and always powerless to cure by ordinary medicine.

A

1. **Abcess**-*Boils*, A collection of puss formed at the expense of the surrounding soft tissues. — Commences with a swelling.

A2 n. C. II. S. baths medicated with C5. El. R. "—" El. J. to the corresponding nerves.

a. *In the breast:* see n° 1, and article *breast.*

b. *In the leg:* see n° 1, also El. R., El. J. or El. B. alternated.

c. *Syphilitic:* see n° 1, also Ven. a. b. s.

d. *In the skull:* see n° 1, c., also El. R. "——" El. J. to the occiput and sympathetic, onct. of C^5 to the part affected.

2. **Abdomen**-*Affections of the belly.*

a. *Ascitcs:* dropsy, effusion of the serous surface of the belly.

SII. a. b. s. El. R. "—" El. J. to the sympath.

b. *Enteritis:* intestinel inflammation,

S II a. b. s. or C II. Baths of C5. El. R. "—-—"

El. J. to the symp ; onct. of C5 to the abdomen.

Comp. El. B. to the abdomen. 20 gr. C5.

c. *Mesenteritis:* inflammation and tubercules of the mesenteric glands.

C a b. s. Baths of C5 El. B. to the symp. Comp. El. B. to the belly. 20 gr. of C5 ; onct. of C5 to the abdomen.

d. *Intestinal Consumption.*

S. A. Baths of C5; onct. of C5 to the belly. El. B. to the symp.; compr. El. B. to the belly, 20 gr. C5; comp. C5. Baths of S. — S5 and A2.

e. *Peritonitis:* Inflammation of the peritoneum or envelope of the bowels; it may be symptomatic or essential. Treatment as n°2, d.

f. *Twisting of the bowels:* (colic so called) see d.

g. *Morbid obesity:* see d ; also El. R. "'—" El. J. to the occ., the symp. and the solar plexus; also baths of S., baths of A. onct. F2 to the hypoc. onct. of C5 to the hypoc. onct. of C5 to the head.

h. *Enteralgia:* nervous colic.

S II a. b. s. 20 gr. of S. Baths of C5. Baths of S. El. B. to the symp. onct. of C5 to the symp.

i. *Ascites:* proceeding from alterations in the mesentcric glands.

C II a. b. s. El. B. to the symp., plex. sol., occ. 10 gr. C5, Baths of C5 or S. or A2, Onct. of C5 to the parts most affected.

j. *Pancreatitis:* inflammation of the pancreas (gland of the abdomen).

S II, El. R. and El. J. to the symp. Baths of C5 or S. Onct. of C5 to the part affected.

k. *False pregnancy:* C II, Baths of C5. El. R. "—" El. J. to the sacred nerves and to the symp. 10 g. C5.

l. *Interrupted labour:* see k.

m. *Alterations of the womb* in general: pains, whites, diflicult labours, falling down of, and every cause which deranges woman in this respect is caused by the viciation of the lymph. C. compr. or injections of C5. El. R. "— " El. J to the sacred and crural nerves; baths of C5 or even comp. of C. Baths of S or A2.

n. *Amcnorrhoea* caused by cold after confinement, see. m.

3. **Acne**-Isolated postules, pointed, most frequently, developed on the shoulders and breast bone, followed after disquamation by purplish spots, etc., two varieties are *acne rosacea* affecting the face, and *mentagra* the chin.

S II. A II a. b. s. C, a, b. s. Baths of C5, of S, of A2, of S5. Comp. of C5.

4. **Adenites**-*See glands.*

5. **Alba, dolens**-See articles *blood, veins, phlebitis.*

6. **Albuminuria**-See *urine.*

7. **Alopecia**-Baldness, see *hair.*

8. **Amaurosis**-See *eyes.*

9. **Amenorrhoea**-see n° 20, and article *menses.*

10. **Anasarca**-See *swellings.*

11. **Anoemia**-Poverty of blood, A. S. baths of A2 compr. A2. onct. A2. over the region of the heart, see *green sickness.*

12. **Aneurism**-See *heart.*

13. **Angina pectoris**-Neuralgia of the heart, characterized by sudden, acute and short pain, with anguish, feeble pulse, etc.

A. A2. S. some dry granules of S., compr. of A2. slight applications over the heart with El. A. see *heart, neuralgia.*

14. **Angina**-See *throat.*

15. **Angioitis**-Inflammation of the sanguine *vascular* system (greek *angios,* vessel) with erysipelas, eruptions, etc. A — A2 II. C5. II. Baths of C5. El, A —. Baths of A2.

16. **Antidotes**-Against the use of a wrong remedy is the same remedy, at the 2nd or 3rd dilution. As a general rule, reduce it 1 or 2 degrees lower than that which caused the disturbance. Against excess of a remedy, lemon juice or vinegar.

17. **Anthrax**-See *Carbuncle, Boils.*

18. **Anus**-See *rectum, prolapsus.*

19. **Aphonia**-Loss of the voice, see *voice.*

20. **Appetite**-Loss of. S. a. b. s. El. R. "—" El. J. to the pit of the stomach. Baths of C5.

21. **Apoplexy**-Commences by: falling unconscious, face injected, laborious respiration.—At other times, the attack is preceded by violent pains in the head, or paralysis, at once, strikes half the body.

S. A2. C. Try, here, all the electricities to the occ., symp., plex. sol. to all the nerves of the legs and arms. Baths, onct. of C5. Baths of A2. Baths medicated with El. B.

When the attack is followed by paralysis, repeat the electric applications, persist with S. A. El. R. El. J. or El. A. to the occ., symp., plex. sol, Baths, onct, of C5 or better C. internally with Baths of S. and A2.

22. **Apthae**-Ulceration of the mouth. Little whitish ulcerations on the membrane of the mouth or alimentary canal S. A2 C5. The same in gargles (20 gr. in a glass of water). Baths of C5.

23. **Arthritis**-S. a. b. s. 20 gr. of S. Baths of C5. comp. of A2. over the heart, onct. of F2. to the hypoc. comp. of C5. to the hypoc. Baths of S.

24. **Arm**-Atrophy of the arm with rheumatism. El. R. El. J. to the occ. to the symp., plex. sol., bracheal nerves. Baths. onct. of C5. or baths and onct. of S. or baths and onct. of A2 to the part. Comp. of El. W.

a. *Paralysis* of arm as n° 24.

b. *Dislacing nerve* of arm, see n° 24.

c. *Pains preventing* movement of arm, see nº 24, but generally El. R. is suflieient.

d. *Numbness* of arm, as n° 24, also A. internally.

e. *Inertia* of the hands and arms: see n° 24, frequently removed by El. R. alone.

f. *Semi-ancylosis* of the elbow and wrist: (see n° 24.) also onct. of C5, or S, or A2. to the part affected.

25. **Articular** pains-C. A2. Baths of C5. El. V. onct. over the region of the heart, of A2, or of C5. or onct. of F2, to the hypoc. Verm. internally.

25. **bis Articulations**-Rickets, rickety children. S. C. A. a. b. s. Baths, onct. of C5. Baths of S, El. R. "—" El. J. "—" El. A. to the symp., to plex. sol., to the occ.

26. **Ascarides**-See *worms.*

27. **Ascitis**-See *abdomen.*

28. **Asphixia**-S. a. b. s., or 20 gr. of S., or 20 gr. of A. all at once on the tongue. El. R. "—" El. J. to the symp. plex. sol. occ. Baths of C5. onct. of the same on the pit of the stomach, and over all the head.

Suffocation from drowning. S. a. b. S. El. R. "—" El. J. to the occ. symp., to the temples, to the pit of the stomach. Baths of C5. onct. of the same to the pit of the stomach; comp. *ibid* of C5. 20 gr. of C5. or 20 gr. of A2.

29. **Asthma**-spasmadic uneasiness of the chest, with yawning, oppression, abundant urine, etc.

S. a. b. s. A. a. b. s. If the origin is nervous, El. R. to the pit of the stomach, symp, and plex. sol.; if it is vascular El. A. to the same places.

Baths of C5, onct. of C5, to the symp. If the chest is attacked P. alternated with the preceding.

a. *Catarrhal asthma* as n° 29. in addition P3 II a. b. s.

b. *Asthma* with *arterial hoemorrhage.* A II. A2 II a. b. s. Baths of C5, A2, comp. A2. over the heart.

c. *An asthma* of 2 years standing, removed by a single application of El. R to the pit of the stomach.

d. *Nervous asthma*, of 10 years standing cured by S II a. b. s., and El. R.

e. *Catarrhal asthma* of many years. S II a. b. s. P3., Baths of C5, onct, of A2.

30. **Atrophy**-General or partial of a limb,

S, C5, A2. Baths of C5, of S. of A2. 10 gr. of C5., onct. of F2. to the hypoc, El. R. "——-" El. J. "—" El. A. to the occ., symp., plex. sol. and nerves of the effected member. Baths of El. B. Onct. of C5 to the hypoc. The cures are numerous and very remarkable of cases of atrophy, some congenital, treated and cured in advanced life.

31. **Aversion** to milk-(in infants, suckling.) Give the nurse S. For the infant onct. to the hypoc. of C5.

B

32. **Beard** (loss of)-S. 20 gr. of C5. onct. of same or of S. to parts, C. a b s. When of syphilitic origin, Ven. a. b. s. Baths of C5. onct. of the same. Baths of S., onct. of Ven.

33. **Belly**-See *abdomen.*

34. **Bladder**-*Gravel*, compare *Loins.* S II. A2 II, a b, s., baths of C5., onct. to the hypoc. of F2. Baths of S., of A2. compr. of El. B. to the pubis, perineum, sacred nerves. El.R. "—" El. J. to the symp., occ,, plex. sol., loins, sacred nerves, onct. of C2, of S. of A5. to the pubis.

a. *Cystitis*, inflammation of, and other bladder diseases. (see n° 34.)

b. *paralysis* of bladder, (see n² 34) also injections of El. B.

c. *Wetting the bed*. Retention of urine, voiding drop by drop, (see b.)

d. *Catarrh* of bladder (see n° 34.)

e. *Polypus* of bladder. C. and C5., and as in n° 34, and in same manner for other bladder affections.

Under the influence of our remedies the stone, if calcareous, is dissolved and voided as a gruel, ash coloured, after 20 or 30 days treatment. If the stone is of another nature it requires a longer period, but afterwards passes under the form of a reddish gruel.

35. **Blenorrhagia**-See *Womb*.

36. **Blenorrhoea**-See *Womb-Vagina*.

37. **Blindness**-See *Eyes*.

38. **Blood**-All diseases of the blood, properly called, are caused first by excess, or rather by an abnormal flow of blood towards one point of the economy, to the detriment of the others. Second, by want or poverty of the blood. Congestion is the result in both cases, but it is *active* or there is active hyperhoemia in the case of excess; it is *passive* or there is passive hyperhoemia in the want either of the blood or circulation. In the first, there is congestion, properly called (of the lungs, of the brain, etc.;) in the second case, an obstruction, sanguine *stagnation* (of the lungs, heart, liver, etc., varicose veins. anaemia, green sickness, etc.)

The maladies, arising from excess of blood, should be treated with small doses, second and third dilutions of angioitics and compresses over the heart, made with 2 granules to a spoonful of water of A or A2. The diseases, arising from want of blood or slowness of circulation, ought to be treated with A II. or A2 II. and C II., which it is often necessary to alternate. These diseases are, essentially, the result of a viciation of the lymph; this is why the antiangioitics should be alternated with the anticancerous.

Special diseases proceeding, either from excess or want of blood, are indicated, with their treatment, in the catalogue, under their respective names.

39. Boils and predisposition to abscesses-S. "—-" A. El. R. "—" El. J. to the occ., symp. onct. to the affected part of C5. Baths of S.

a. *on lower eyelids*, El. R. "—-" El. J. to the part affected, onct. C5. or S. or A2. Comp of S. or A2.

b. *On upper eyelids:* as above, also onct. or compr. of S5.

40. Bowels-Flatulence of, rumbling noise of:-(see *stomach*).

41. Bowels (diseases of)-S. II a b. s. C. II. a b. s. C5. a b. onct. of C5. to the abdomen. Baths, comp., onct. of C5. of S. Pass lightly some drops of El. B. with the hand over the abdomen. El. B. "—" El. J. to the symp., occ., plex. sol., pit of the stomach.

a. Intestinal *consumption*. C. II a b. s. (See 41).

b. *Mesentiritis* (See a).

c. *Tubercles* of mesenteric gland (See a), also 20 gr. of C. or C5. daily, alternating the dry granules with the diluted remedies.

d. *Polypus of the Bowels*. C. a. b. s. C5. a. b. s. S. a. b. s., Baths of C5., S., A2., S5. El. R. "—-" El. J. to pit of the stomach, symp. and bottom of the spine. Onct. of C5. or S. El. B. to affected parts.

e. *strangulation* of the bowels. S. a. b. s. El R, "—" El. J. to the symp., plex. sol. Baths, onct., compr. of C5. or S. Comp. El. B., 20 gr. of-C2. and compr. of A2. to the part.

f. *Weakness* of bowels. S. a b. s. Baths of C5. of S., of A2. compr. of El. B. El. R. "—" El. J. to the symp., plex. sol. and the sides of the spine. 28 gr. of C5. or of S 5.

g. *Colic* of bowels (See f). and *Colics.*

h. *Rumbling noise of bowels* (See f).

i. *Periodical inflammation of bowels:* F2 a b. s. 20 gr. of C5. (See f).

42. Brain (softening of)-See also *Rickets.* Onct. to the whole of the head of C5. A". and S5.

43. Breast diseases of, congestion etc. CII. C2 II. a b. s. El. B. to plex. sol. and symp., baths of C5. C. S5. El.R. to plex. sol. and to symp.

a. *Abscess* of breast, arrested by C. II "—" A2 II. a b. s.

b. *Cracked nipples.* S. C5. onct., compr., baths of C5. S. S5. Comp. El. B. or El. R. S2. a b. s. compr. of S5. or C5. Ven. a b. s.

c. *Inflammation of the nipple* (See above b.)

d. *Chapped nipples.* (See b.), but first apply CII a. b. s. compr. and onct. of same.

e. *Loss of milk* caused by sudden anger. Cure of a woman aged 26 years-In general give C2. a b. s. El. R. to the symp., plex. sol. C5. a. b. s. Baths of C5.

f. *Secretion of milk at an abnormal period.* Galac torrhoea.

See *Milk, flow of.*

44. Breath, (fetidity of)-See *Mouth.*

45. Bronchitis-See Lungs.

46. Bubo-See Syphilis.

47. Burns and Scalds-Grave, with sores, as n° 24. See also *wounds gangrenous.*

C

48. **Calculus**-See *Bladder, Loins.*

49. **Cancer and Scirrhus**-This serious and hitherto incurable disease, is characterized: lst by the evolution of cancerous tissue, in one or many parts of the economy ; 2nd by the easy reproduction of affections which have been removed or destroyed; 3rd by the frequent development of a special class of cachexy. The *cancerous tissue* is a morbid product without analogy, organized, extending, by the disorganization and transformation of the surrounding tissues, into its own substance and ulcerating indefinitely. (Jousset.) We have stated, during 20 years, *the radical cure of cancer:* the doctors, saving some honorable exceptions, continue to kill persons, affected with cancer, by opium.

There will be found, in our pamphlets, especially in: *Un poco di storia sui rimedi Mattei*, numerous proofs of the fact that we here advance ; there will, also, be found curious anecdotes of doctors who hold on to opium and obstinately refuse to work miracles by the anti-cancerous of electrohomeopathy. Their conduct merits to be exposed to the public, who will end by judging the men, whose mission it is to cure.

Treatment. C. or C4. or C5. — A. or A2; baths of C5. compr. of C5. onct. of C 5, to the part. Baths, onct., compr. of A2. Baths of S. or S5. — El. R. "—" El. J. to the corresponding nerves.

When there is a wound, El. V. or El. B. or onct. C5., onct. of F2. to the hypoc. also baths medicated by the white, green, red, or angioitic electricities.

a. *Cancer* of the stomach: as n° 49.

b. *Cancer* of the bowels: as n° 49.

c. *Cancer* of the tongue: as n° 49; also gargles, of C., of A., of El. B. of C5. of C4, of S.

d. *Cancer* of the eyelids : as n° 49., also comp. of El. B. and onct. of S.

e. *Cancer* of the nose : as n° 49., also inhalations of C. of A, of El. B. or El. V. onct, of C5, or of S., or of S5. A2 to the exterior, surface of the nose.

f. *Cancer* of the breast : as n° 49.

g. *Cancer* of the womb : as n° 49., also injections of C. of A2. El. B. or El. V. and onct, of C5. to the pubis and sacred nerves. El. R. and El. J. to the sacred nerves. 20 gr. of C5.

h. *Cancer* of the anus : as n° 49.

i. *Cancer* of the lips: as n° 49, generally it is detached and comes away, in a single piece, when the remedy has sufiiciently penetrated the system.

j. *Cancer* of the Pylorus ; as n° 49.

k. *Cancer* Fungous tumours of the breast; treated as n° 49, g. A tumour of this class in the breast, operated on already several times, with offensive suppuration, frequent heamorrhage, shooting pains, etc., has been seen to come away in fragments.

l. *Cancer Ulcerated cancer of the Vulva:* treated as n° 49, g.

m. *Cancer Fistulvus ulcers of the anus:* treated as n° 49, g.

Madame Albine Massotti, afflicted with cancer of the womb, was under treatment during 8 years, in three hospitals of Bologna, without result. I cured her in 14 months; no reappearance of disease 12 years after : this patient is still alive.

Remarks-The larger the wound, the greater the difiiculty of cure ; at too advanced a stage, it becomes frequently impossible and the remedies can only sooth it. But, on the other hand, why allow the disease to develop itself? I understand that the classic routine was obliged to allow its development and growth, in order to be able to amputate it : but it does nothing to ward off the evil during the time that it is yet curable.

50. **Cancer** or **chancre syphilitic**-See *syphilis.*

51. **Caries of the bones**-Follow the treatment n° 49.

At this moment, a *new remedy*, appearing to have a very special action on caries, is undergoing trial.

a. *Of the teeth* (decayed teeth), as n° 49, also gargles with the internal remedies, there mentioned, and onct. of C5 to the jaws.

b. *Of the bones of the nose*, as n° 49, also inhalations of C. and C5. onct. of C5. to the diseased part.

52. **Carbuncle**-C. a b. s compr. of C. or C5. or onct., Baths of C5. or baths, onct., comp. of S. comp. A2. El. R. and El. J. to the corresponding nerves, S.

If not stopped, death will follow in the course of 24 hours.

53. **Catalepsy**-El. R. to the occ. and symp. dissipates it in a few seconds; if it persists C. II a. b. s. Baths, onct of C5. to the occ. Baths of El. B.

54. **Cataract**-See *eyes.*

55. **Catarrh**-See *lungs.*

56. **Change of life**-S. II. a. b. s. see also *womb. menses.*

57. **Chill**-Taking cold, and its consequences. Arrest the fever by F. onct. of C5. to the hypoc. comp. to the head of El. B. El. R. "—" El. J. to the occ. and symp. S. II . a b. s. 20 gr. of C5 baths of C5.

a. *Stiff neck.* El. R. "—" El. J. to the nerve, comp. El. B. onct. of S. of A2. Comp. Baths, onct. of C5. S.

58. **Chicken pox**-See *fevers.*

59. **Chlblains**-Can be generally dispersed with S. or 20 gr. of S. or onct. of C5 Baths or comp. of C5. Baths, comp., onct. of S. or comp. El. R. or El. B. onct. of F2 to the hypoc.

60. **Chlorosis**-See *anemia, green sickness.*

61. **Cholera**-Preservative, in time of an epidemic: 20 gr. of S. during the day. At the onset, 20 gr. at at once of S. dry, or S. a b. s. El. R. El. J. to the occ. and especially to pit of the stomach and the symp.

If the disease is obstinate, Baths of C5 or A3 or El. B.

Consequences of cholera. S. a. b. s. El. R, "—" El. J . to the occ., symp., plex. sol. Baths of C5. A2 of S: Comp. F2 to the hypoc.

62. **Chorea**-See *St. Vitus's dance.*

63. **Clap**-See *Syphilis.*

64. **Colic**-S. a. b. s. or 20 gr. of S. El. R. "—" El. J. to pit of the stomach, to the symp. Baths of C5 onct. of C5 to pit of the stomach, C5 or 10 gr. C5. onct. and comp. of F2 to the pit of the stomach.

64. **bis. Colds in the head**-S. a. b. s. onct. comp. of S. C5 or baths of C5.

The predisposition to take cold disappears with the prolonged use of antiscorofoloso.

For stopping in the nose, touch the base of the nose with El. R.—See also *Chills.*

65. **Coma**-See *lethargy.*

66. **Condyomota**-See *tumors.*

67. **Congestion of blood vessels with constipation**-See *Frost-bitten.* Also onct. to the whole of the head and face with C5 comp. Baths and onct. of A2.

68. **Congestions** of all kinds, either of glands or tissues; C. II. a b. s. Baths of C5., or C5. II a b. s. Baths of El. R., El. R. "—" El. J. to the corresponding nerves. Baths of C.

Congestion of the liver or spleen, F. II a b. s. or 10 gr. of the same. Onct. of F2. or C5. or F. to the hypoc. Baths of C5. El. R. "—" El. J. to plex. sol , symp. occ., hypoc. Baths of A2.

69. **Contraction** of the **hand** from wounding the nerve. S a b. s. El. R. "—" El J. to the nerves of the hand. Baths, onct., compr., of C5. Onct. or compr. of S. or El. B.

70. **Convulsions**-According to the case whether they proceed from worms, itch, or defective circulation, they are treated with: Verm. II. S. II. or C5. II. A II. to be taken frequently.

a. *During summer*, as n° 70, also baths C5.

b. *From fright*, S. II . El. R. to the symp.

c. *Convulsive movements*. Baths of C5.S II. El. R. "—" El. J. Baths of El. B.

d. *Convulsions and germs* of insanity; treated as c.

e. *convulsions* with itching of the nose. Verm. II. Baths of C5. Onct. of F2. to the hypoc. Baths of El. B.

f. *Convulsions* from alterations in the sympathetic nerve; from fright ; treated as c relieved by a single application of El. R,

g. *Nervous alterations* from the effects of carbonic acid gas.— As letter c.

h. *convulsions* left by cholera, treated as c. also onct. of A2 to the region of the heart. Onct. or compr. of F2. to the hypoc. or baths of S.

i. *convulsions* during the menses A2 III. and baths of C5 or. of A2.

71. **Corns**-S. C5. Onct., baths, or compr. of C5. Onct. of S. Compr. of El. R. or of El. B.

72. **Coryza**-Cold in the head; S. onct. of C5. to the head. baths of the same. onct. of S. El. R. "—" El. J. to the occ. symp. El. B. It has been cured with a few granules of S. or C5.

73. **Coxalgia**-See *Hips.*

74. **Cough**-See *lungs.*

75. **Cramp of the stomach**-Often removed instantly by giving 10 gr. of S. dry, at once, in a single dose. El. R., El. J, to the symp., plex. sol., occ.

a. *Menstrual cramp*; as 75, also El. A. A II. compr. of A2. to the painful part and over the heart.

b. *Of the legs:* cured by onct. of C5. or baths, compr. of C5. S. C5. comp. of El. B.

c. *Of the back of the head:* El. R. "—" El. J. to the occ. or onct, of C5. of S. of A2. El. B.

d. *Of the hands* (writers cramp). Onct. of C5 or of S., El. B. (see letter c).

e. *In the nerve of the heel:* El. R. removes this instantly, (see d.). In case of returns baths of C5.

76. **Croup**-Cases have been cured, in a few minutes, by gargles of El. R. or El. B. "—" El. J. to the occ. little hypoglosses. F. II. onct. of F2. or C5. to the hypoc. or baths or C5. P. gargles of El. B.

77. **Cystites**-See *Bladder.*

78. **Cutaneous diseases**-Eruptions on the skin of a thousand varieties. S. A. C5. S5. El. R. "—" El. J. to the symp., occ., plex. sol. or baths, onct. and comp. of C5 S. S5. or A2. Compr. or onct. either of C5, or F2 . to the hypoc. But the most eflicacious is generally the bath of C5.

a. *Eruptions*- which reappeared during 16 years cured by the means indicated.

b. The same for eruptions on the lower part of the abdomen.

c. Also Impetigo on the face in a man 25 years of age.

d. *Herpes with severe angioitis*; as n° 78; but the antiangioitics and El. A are preferable.

e. *Herpes furfuracea* on the head: as n° 78. persists with onct, of C5. and of S.

f. *Squamus eruption* over the entire body; baths of C5. of S. 20 gr. of C. or of C5. (See also n° 78).

g. *Exanthema* of the hands, as letter e.

h. *Eruptions* with thread worms at same time combined with treatment n° 78. a *vermifuge* at 1st dilution.

79. **Curvature of the spine**-See *Spine.*

D

80. **Deafness** and difficulty of hearing.

If the cause is nervous: S. C". a b. s. onct, to the entire ear of C5., of S. El. R. in the ear. Baths of S5. El. R. "—" El. J. to the occ.,symp., at the back and root of the ear by opening the mouth. Compr. of El. B. to all the nerves of the ear.

If the origin is congestive A. A2 a b. s. compr., onct. of A2. to the ear. Baths of A2. of C5. of El. A. compr. of El. A. to the ear, Onct. of A2. to the heart.

a. *Deafness* of 30 years standing cured by El. R. alone.

b. *Ditto*, of 30 years cured with A. alone internally and externally.

c. *Ditto*, of 8 years with S. alone internally and externally.

d. *Ditto*, complete and chronic cured with C5. internally and externally.

81. **Debility in general**-S. Baths of C5. El. R. "—" El. J. to the symp., plex. sol., occ., and all the nerves of the face and body. By these means have been treated: weakness of the hand, following a fracture: weakness of the arm, of the sight, of the brain, bowels, debility from prolonged lactation, etc.

This treatment should be followed, for all debility in general, saving possible variations in the application of the electricities to the affected nerves, variations which must be left to individual judgment.

82. **Delirium**-See *fevers.*

83. **Delirium tremens**-Same treatment as indicated for *debility* n° 81. But employ preferably the antiscrofulous.

84. **Derbyshire neck**- See *glands.*

85. **Diabetes**-Abundant secretion of sugary urine, accompanied with a peculiar cachexy, characterized by tendancy to formation of tubercles and to gangrene. S. C. A. Baths of C5 or A2. El. R. El. J. or El. A. to symp., plex. sol., occ., and sides of the spine. Onct. of C5 or F2 to the hypoc. Baths of S., 20 gr of S5. See also *urine.*

86. **Diarrhoea, dysentery**-If no blood is passed: S. or 20 gr. of S. Baths of S. El. R. "—" El. J. to the symp., to pit of the stomach, and plex. sol. Baths of C5.

If there is blood: A. or 20 gr. of A2, or A2 first dilution, or El. A. to the pit of the stomach. Onct. of C5 to the symp. or of F2 to the hypoc. Baths, onct. of A2 to the region of the heart, Baths of C5.

87. **Digestion** difficult-Dyspepsia-S. or 20 gr. of S. or baths of C5. El. R. to the pit of the stomach.

More numerous or more certain results cannot be found.

88. **Disturbanccs of the head**-See *head.*

89. **Dysmenorrhoea**-See *menses.*

90. **Dyspepsia**-See *digestion.*

91. **Dysentery**-See *diarrhoea.*

92. **Dysuria**-See *urine, bladder.*

93. Drowning. Recovery from-See *Asphyazia*.

94. Dropsy-Attention must be paid to the cause and the treatment modified accordingly.

Of the womb. C III. a b. s. compr. of C5.

Of the abdomen. F III. a b. s. compr. of F2 to the hypoc. El. B. to plex. sol., sym. occ.

Of the heart. A2 III. a b. s. comp. of A2 (2 granules) to the heart.

Baths of C5. S5. S. El. R. "—" El. J. to plex. sol. symp.

a. *Dropsy in general*, n° 94. Persist strongly with the electricities to the occ. symp. plex. sol., onct. of F2 to the hypoc. also of C5. F II a b. s. S. II. a b. s. or C II ab. s. or A2. a b. s.

E

95. Ears (Diseases of)-Ear-ache-S. S5. C. A2. a b. s. onct. comp. to the ears of C5. S. A2. Comp. of El. B. to the entire ear. El. R. El. J. to the little muscles which are behind the ear and to the root of the ear, at its junction with the jaw, (by opening the mouth). Baths of C5 S. A2. El. B. in the ear.

a. *Otitis*, inflammation of the ear, as 95.

b. *Otorrhoea*, discharge from the ear, as 95.

c. *Otorrhoea*, with toothache, as n° 95.

And onct. comp. of C5. to the painful point externally.

d. *Dysecia*, weakness of hearing, as n° 95.

e. *With congestion*: A. or A2 a b. s. Baths, onct., comp. of A2. El. A. or El. B. to the entire ear.

f. *Noises or buzzing in the ear*: El. A. to the occ. symp., to the muscles behind the ear, to the root of the ear (in opening the mouth) a few drops of El. A. if there is congestion, or as n° 95, if not congested.

g. *Hemorrhage* from the ear, A II or A2 II. a b s. comp. of A. or A2. to the heart. El. A. to the occ., symp., and slight application over the heart. Comp., onct., baths of A2. It has also been relieved by S. C. C5., the last especially. Onct., comp. (to the heart) and baths of C5.

h. *Inflammation* of the salivary glands under the ear (parotiditis) C. II C5 a b. s. 20 gr. of C5. onct., compr. of C5, to the affected part, Baths, onct. of C5. to the hypoc. El. B. in compr. El R. "—" El. J. around the swelling.

i. *Polypus in the auditory canal*: El. B. in the ear, with 20 gr. of C5. Baths, onct. compr of C5. Injections in the ear of C5. C. a b. s. El. R. in the ear and applied to the three little muscles behind, or injections of S5. or S. or A2.

j. *Spasms in the ear*: El. R. or El. B. in compresses, (see n° 95.)

k. *Otorrhoea* caused by suppression of milk: cured with S. and compresses of the same.

96. Ecchymosis of the Eyes-(Black Eye) A. A2, compresses of C5. El. A. to the occ., to super and sub orbital nerves; to symp. onct. of A2. Baths or compresses of El. B.

97. Ecthyma-Large roundish pustules-(See *cutaneous diseases*).

98. Eczema-Hot, burning pustules. S. A. onct., baths, comp. C5, or onct., baths, comp. of S5, El. R. "—" El. J. to the symp., occ., plex. sol. Baths of S. or onct. of C5. to the hypoc, compr. of El. B.

99. Elephantiasis-Diseases of the lymphatic vessels, accompanied with swelling of the lower extremities, commencing at the groin, and extending progressively until the leg, monstrously enlarged, effaces the jutting out of the foot.

C. S. A. A2. C5. Baths, onct., comp. of C5. or S5. or S. Compr. El. V. or of R. or J. or of C, El. R. "-—-" El. J. to the corresponding nerves, and to symp., occ., plex. sol., or baths onct., comp. of A2. Onct. and comp. of F2. to the hypoc.

A woman, aged 60 years, suffering from Elephantiasis of the left leg, was cured with these compresses only.

100. Epilepsy-A nervous disease, manifesting itself by convulsive movements, and complete loss of sense and hearing.

It is not always easy to recognize the cause, therefore it is better to regard the probable causes, viz : *The circulation, worms or scrofula* and to treat it in consequence. A, or A2. verm: S. or C, *the third dilution, of which 10 teaspoonfuls will be given daily*. The fits are not announced, but symptoms of uneasiness and vertigo, sometimes precede them. After the fits, stupor.

101. Eplstaxis-Bleeding from the nose, A. or A2. a b. s. generally arrest it. If the internal remedies do not suffice, employ inhalations of A or A2. or baths, or onct., comp. over the heart of this same remedy.

102. Eruptions-See *Fevers*.

103. Erysipelas-El. R. to the occ. at the onset, frequently averts an attack, S II or 5 g. of the same S5. comp. or baths of C5.

a. If the complaint returns, persist with El. R. to the occ., to the sub orbital (when the face is attacked) to the super orbital, to the symp. comp. El. B. or El. R. "—" El. J. to the face.

b. Phlegmonous erysipelas in right arm with vertigo. A II A2 II. baths of C5. or of A2. comp. of. El. B. or A.

c. Periodical erysipelas. F. "—" A., baths of C5. Onct. of F2. to the hypoc. comp. of El. B. baths, onct., comp. of A2 .

d. Erysipelas with oedema in leg. see c. also onct. of A2. baths of C5, persist with these two last.

106. Excoriations severe of the penis-Ven. compr. baths of C5. or S. or baths, onct. comp. of S. comp. El. R. El. R. "—" El. J. to sacred nerves.

107. Excressences fleshy-Compare *Tumours* letter a. and Syphilis if it is a question of syphiitic vegetation. Apart from these cases treat with S. C5. compr. or onct. of C5. or of S. or A2. baths of S5.

108. Eyes. Sight-Affections of the sight.

a. *Weakness of the sight*, or ambliopia. This is frequently the beginning of amaurosis. El. R. to the occ., to sub and super orbitals with S. or A a b. s. 20 gr. of C5. compr. to the entire head of El. B. onct., compr. to the head of C5., baths of C5. onct. of S. or A3. to the sub and super orbitals. El. R. "—" El. J. to occ., symp., sub and super orbitals, forehead, root of nose. Baths of A2. S. or El. B.

b. *Opthalmia*, or diseases of the eye- In opthalmia a powerful resource is found in electricities, applied to the occiput, to the sympathetic, the sub and super orbital nerves, the base of the nose, the forehead and temples. The remedies indicated at the commencement of the number apply to opthalmia whether *catarrhal granular, vascular, congestive*, etc.

For syphilitic opthalmia: Ven. II. a b s, baths, compr. and onct. with Ven. and other remedies as n° 108. The cures already afl'ected of all classes of opthalmia are innumerable. Many were recently cured with *antiscrofoloso nuovo or* 2.

Instantaneous results are not rare here. In cases where the disease is obstinate it is necessary to attack it, in preference, with the anticancerous, among which C. C2. C5 succeed the best.

c. *Cataract*-Formation of opaque membranes which cover the organ of sight. Remedies indicated above, and more, persist with baths of C5 S. A2. lotion of the same to the whole head, and of F2. or C5. to the hypoc.

N. B.-When the cataract commences to fall off, which happens after 30 or 40 days of treatment, the eyes must be shaded from the light exactly the same as after the operation.

d. *Staphyloma*-Transparent or opaque tumour formed either on the cornea, the sclerotic or on the iris; it is a scrofulous product as well as cataract. Follow treatment indicated n° 108 at letter c., not forgetting onct. of F2. to the hypoc. During the night may be applied, advantageously, to the closed eye, compr. of S. or C5. A2. S5. C. and A.

In a shorter or longer period, according to the humour to combat, the cornea is cleansed and recovers its transparency.

e. *Venereal staphyloma*-Ven. compr. of Ven. on the closed eye. (See d).

f. *Specks in the cornea*-(See d).

g. *Hemorrhage of the eyes*-A II. A2 II. a b. s. onct. to the head of A2. of C5., baths of C5. El. A. to occ., symp. and all the nerves of the head. Onct. of F2. or C5. to the hypoc.

h. *Strabismus, squinting*-See n° 108, I once cured it by a single application of red electricity.

i. *Ecchymoses*-(See this word).

j. *Small tumours at edge of eyelids*-(See 108).

k. *Bleared eyes*-See n° 108. and besides comp. on the closed eye with A. or A2. and the white or angioitic electricities.

l. *Albinos*-Inability to support the light. Sometimes it is sufficient to once apply El R. to symp., sub. and supor orbital. occ., forehead ; also well to use El. R. "—" El. J. to points aforesaid. Compr. to the head of El. B. or onct. of C5. S. or A2. (See 108).

m. *Amaurosis*, dimness of vision-as l. Cures are known of cases arrived at almost total blindness.

n. *Indistinct vision*-cured by a single application of El. R.

o. *Shortness of sight*-and almost loss, (the patient not distinguishing objects) consequence of percussion, disease of 3 years standing: man aged 78 years cured by first application of El. R. to sub. and super orbitals.

p. *Eyes burnt by lunar caustic*-Compr. of El.B., S. internally. Compr. of C5 and other remedies above indicated.

Also cured by these means : eye displaced from its orbit by syphilis.

Eye displaced by an enormous staphyloma. Chronic opthalmia of 27 years.

Cornea split. Retraction of the eye. Sight troubled during 27 years.

Loss of sight during the night. Opthalmia complicated with cataract. A complete cataract on the right eye, and one half formed on the left eye of same individual. Weakness of the eyes. Case of complete blindness, etc. There is enough to fill a book if all the cures were enumerated.

109. Eyelids-Inflammation of; SII . CII. a. b. s. compresses of these remedies, of El. B. and El. R. "—" El. J. to the occ., symp., sub and super orbitals, forehead and base of nose. Baths, onct., compr. of C.

a. *Paralysis of:* n° 109. Comp. of El. R. to the eye lids.

b. When there is severe inflammation baths of C5. S. and A repeated.

c. *Spasms of, with vertigo:* A. II. A2. II. C2. a b. s. compr. of these remedies to super orbital, El. B. to occ., symp, and sub. orbitals.

F

110. Face-Rheumatic pains of. El. R "—-" Fl. J. or compr. El. B.; onct., compr., or baths of C5. onct. of S. or S5. S. 20 gr. C5. A II a b. s.

a. *Congestive pains of* (caused by flow of blood to the head) A2 II onct. to the entire head of C5. or A2. Compresses with A. or A2. over the region of the heart (5 gr. 10 spoonfuls of water.)

b. *Paralysis of:* See *Paralysis.*

c. *Inflammatory tubercles* on the face. S. C5. onct., compr. Baths of C5. of S. Baths of S5. El. R. "—" El. J. to symp., plex. sol., occ., sub orbital; onct. C5. to the hypoc.

d. *Lupus*-First shows itself as livid, solitary and indolent tubercles followed by purulent ulcers, etc. It appears to attack the face in preference.

C. C5. A2. comp., baths of C5. or S. comp. of El. B. El. R. "—" El. J. to the symp., occ., sub and super orbital, to base of nose, temples and forehead. Onct. of C5. or F2. to the hypoc. but especially baths and compr. of C5.

e. *Impetigo of the face:* chronic eruption of pustules, more or less close together, the summit of which soon suppurates forming large crusts, scattered or united ; treatment as letter d.

f. *Acne of the nose:* as letter: e.

g. *Blemishes of the face:* (liver spot.) F, onct. or compr. of F2. or F. to the hypoc. or C5. El R. "—" El. J. to the occ. and all the nerves of the face.

h. *Permanent erysipelas of the face*, cured: See d.

111. Fainting Fits-Arrested with 10 gr. S. given all at once dry on the tongue.

112. Falling sickness-See *epilepsy.*

113. Favus-See *Scald head.*

114. Feet-(Excessive perspiration of.) S. A. Baths of C5. S. A2. of El. B. onct. of F2 to the hypoc. El. R. "—" El. J. to the symp., plex. sol. and nerves of the legs.

a. *contusion of the foot* of 8 years standing cured by El. R. alone. See 114.

b. *Pain in the instep* caused by bone out of place. See 114.

c. *Swelling of foot:* S. A2. a b. s. El. B. baths of C5. S. A2. El. R. "—" El. J. to the nerves of the foot, especially under the hollow of the foot.

115. Fevers-All fevers are treated by F. internally and F2 to the hypoeondra in compresses or onctions.

The more violent the fever the more the remedy should be diluted, and the more dilute, the more frequently it must be given, for example, a tea spoonful every five minutes if possible.

Electricities may also be applied to the occiput, alternating the red with the yellow; the white may also be employed alone.

Sometimes, fever is only the result of defect in the circulation, or change in the blood. The angioitics, in restoring the blood, to its normal condition, counteract fever ; reciprocally the febrifuges, which are always beneficial in cases of fever from any cause, act in restoring the normal circulation.

a. *Typhoid fever* F. III a b. s. onct. to the hypoc. of F. or C5.

Nervous fever F. II a b. s. alternate onct. to the hypoc. of F2. C5.

Mucous fever F II a b. s. alternate onct. to the hypoc. of F2. C5.

Bilious fever F II a b. s. alternate onct. to the hypoc. of F2 C5.

Catarrhal fever F. a b. s. alternate onct. of F2. C5 and P3 II El. R. to symp., plex. sol. and sides of the seventh vertebra.

Milk fever P II "—" C II a b. s.

b. *Intermittent fever ague.* F 1st dilution.

Begin to take it in 10 or 15 times, during the day, whilst the fever is not present and continue afterwards.

Pernicious fever: F II a b. s. onct. of F2 to the hypoc. or, better still, of F.

Inflammatory fever in general: F II a b. s.

Feverish symptoms of short duration: F. onct. to the hypoc. of F. and C5.

Scarlatina: F. "—" S. will facilitate the eruption ; the same applies to all eruptive fevers, nettle rash, measles, miliary fever, small pox, etc.

In some cases white electricity to the occ. does good. Eruptions that have reentered are treated and cured by scrofoloso 1st dilution alone.

c. The consequences left by fevers, cachexy, debility, exhaustion, etc. are cured by S. a b. s. onct. of F2 to the hypoc. baths of C5 El. R. "—" E. J. to all the nerves. onct. of C5 to the hypoc.

116. Fistula-Originating in scrofola, treated with anti scrofolous and anti-cancerous, comp. or baths of C5. baths of S. A2 El. R. "—" El. J. to the corresponding nerves.

a. *Dental fistula.* See 116. comp. of C5.

Fistula of the anus. S. baths, comp., onct. of C5 comp. of El. B. of A2.

b. *Stercorous fistula* of the right groin.

Of seven years standing cured as n° 116, but continually baths of C5.

c. Cure also of 20 fistulas of the anus and scrotum in a man of 48 years. — S. C. C5. Baths and onctions as indicated n° 116, and also b.

d. *Fistula of the gum,* O. "—" A2. gargles of C5. of C. of El. B. onct. of C5. to the exterior of the jaw.

117. Fractures-Even complicated. S. II. comp., onct., baths of S. or C5. or S5. Comp. of El. A; El. R. " —" El. J. to the corresponding nerves. El. B.

118. Frost bites-Blue color of the face caused by cold. A. A2. El. A. to occ. symp. Baths onct., or comp. of A2. to the face, or baths of C5. and onct. of F2 to the hypoc. 20 gr. of C5.

a. With perpetual chill: C. El. R. "—" El. J. Baths of C5. or S. onct. of F2. to the hypoc. Baths of El. B. or of S5.

b. *Foot frozen* and twisted: treatment as preceding.

c. Man, frozen by falling into a well and remaining there during the night, was cured by these means.

119. Furuncles-See *Boils.*

G

120. Galactorrhoea-See *Milk.*

121. Ganglionitis-Inflammation of the lymphatic ganglions; little knots in the course of the nerves and lymphatic vessels, formed by the interlacing of ligaments united by the cellular tissue. C II C5. II 10 gr. of C. Baths, onct., comp. of C5. El. R. "—" El. J. to the corresponding nerves. Comp. of El. B, or S, or A2.

122. Gangrene-C. II a b. s. or 20 gr. of C5. Baths, onct., compr. of C5. Baths of S. El. R. "—" El. J. to corresponding nerves. Compr. of El. B. or El. V. onct. of S5.

Numerous cases of gangrene have been cured by this treatment. Humid gangrene from gunshot wounds, gangrene of extremities caused by dropsy, gangrene of foot resulting from a wound and which it was decided to amputate; another case where the foot was already black ; gangrene following an ancient amputation of the arm etc.

123. Gastralgia, Gastritis-See *stomach.*

124. Generation (organs of)-Spermatorrhoea. S II. C II A II a b. s. El. R. " —" El. J. to the sacred nerves, to perineum, pubis, occ., symp; baths, onct. (to sacrum, pubis, perineum) of C5. S. onct. of A2 to the above mentioned parts. Baths of El. B. 20 gr. of C5.

125. Glands-Adenitis or inflammation of the glands; also little fleshy tumours, hard, indolent, without alteration of the color of the skin developed on the course of the tendons.

The remedies, indicated here, apply to adonitis, which is alteration of the glands properly so called, also to the tumours above mentioned.

C. S. C5. and A II alternated with remedies indicated n° 121. Baths, onct., compr., of C5 or S. comp. El. B. El. R. "—" El. J. to the corresponding nerves.

a. *Mesenteric glands* C II a b. s. see n° 125.

b. *Fatty congestion* of the whole glandular and vascular system (leprosy). C II a b. s. 20 gr. of C5. A2. "—" C II a. b. s. See n° 125.

c. *Tyroid gland.* (When on the throat). 125, also: El. R "—" El. J. to the base of the gland, comp. El. B onct. of C5 or of S.

d. *Parotid glands.* Inflammation of the salivary glands under the ear. C II a b. s. comp. gargles of C5. El. R. "—" El. J. to corresponding nerves, A.

e. *Swollen glands* of the neck, not suppurating: see n° 125. Comp. El. A. El. B.

126. Gonorrhoea-See *Syphilis.*

127. Gout, Arthritis-Acute: S. or S2 or S5. in 2nd dilutions. A2 II Baths, onct., comp. of C5 or S. S5. onct of F2 to the hypoc. or C5 comp. El. B. El. R. "—" El. J. to the occ., symp., plex. sol. to the painful nerves. But especially baths of C5 or El. B. (two spoonfuls in the bath) or else 20 gr. C. or C5.

a. *Chronic* as n°. 127, but given at the first dilution.

b. *Hand contracted by the gout*, as 127 treat especially by external means.

128. Gravel-See *Bladder.*

129. Green sickness (Chlorosis anemia) especially shown by the lips, gums and tongue, A. C. a b. s. S. 20 gr. of C5. gargle of El. B. El. R. to the symp., occ., plex. sol. Baths of A2. onct. of F2 to the hypoc.

Other symptoms of chlorosis are headaches with palpitations of the heart, swelling of the legs, suppression or abnormal state of the menses, sadness, tears, anxiety, peevishness. A II. C. C5. a b. s. comp. or onct. to the heart of A2. or baths of A2. El. B. to occ., symp., plex. sol.

130. Gums (Disorders of the). S. C. A2. C5 or 10 gr. of C5 gargles with all these remedies or with El. R. El. B. or El. A.

131. Hair (Loss of). S. A. Baths of C5 onct., comp. of C5 to the head, baths, onct. compr. of S. El. R. "—" El. J. to occ , symp., to little hypoglossids, to super orbital, and temples. Wash the head with El. B.

131. bis. Haemorrhage of all kinds. Arrested by the angioitics, alternated sometimes with S II. C II. a b. s. El. A. or B.

a. (of the womb) A II or A2 II a b. s. comp. to the heart of A. or A2. Baths, onct., comp. of A2. Baths of C5 onct. of F2 to the hypoc.

132. Head-The points selected to act on the whole of the head with electricities, are : the occiput, little hypoglossids, temples, sub and super orbitals, forehead and base of the nose. Touch also the two sides of the seventh cervical vertebra.

a. *Cephalagia-Headache*-El. B. to occ., little hypogl. seventh servical vertebra. Moisten lightly the head with El. B. Onct. to head and neck of C5 S. A2 El. R. to little hypogl. El. R. "—" El. J. to the occ., temples, symp. El. R. or El. A. to the entire head.

b. If the headache is congestive: El. A to the points above indicated ; compr., onct. of A2 to the head and neck; baths of A2 . Onct of F2 to the hypoc, compr. of A2 to the region of the heart.

c. If proceeding from derangement or affections of the womb: C II a b. s, onct. of C5 to the head. Baths of C2. 20 gr. of C5. El. B. to the arch of the foot.

d. *Congestive face-ache.* See b.

e. *Encephalitis.* S. II a b. s. See a.

f. *Menengitis, acute Cephalo-menengitis;* inflammation of the coveringof the brain, C II a b. s. and see: e.

g. *Hydrocephalus or dropsy of the brain:* A2. II a b. s. If tubercles exist C. a b. s. See b. for the rest.

For infants suckling give the nurse S. A2. a b. s. to the infant the remedies indicated letter b.

h. *Tubercles of the brain*, C. II A II a b. s. compr. of El. B. onct., compr. (to brain) and baths of C5 or S. compr., onct. of C. El. R "— " El. J. to occ., symp, and all the nerves of the head, onct., compr. to the hypoc. of C5 F2. Onct., compr. to the head of A2.

i. *Softening of the brain.* See h.

j. *Commotion of the brain.* S. A. a b. s. and see h.

k. *Headache* and other pains in the head recurring periodically. F. a b. s. onct. to hypoc. of F2 and C5. see also a.

We have already stated that the febrifuges are specific in every case of periodical disease.

l. *Ordinary headache* is removed by the electricities alone El. R. "—-" El J. to occ., symp., compr. of El. B.

m. *Weariness*, fatigue of the head. See l.: S. internally and baths, onct., compr. of S. of C5. baths of El. B. or El. R.

n. A cephalgia declared incurable, accompanied with torpor, was removed by a single application of El. B. to the sub and super orbitals.

Another case of 8 month's standing, cured instantly. Pain caused by tubercles in the brain removed by El. R. alone.

Idem caused by excess of brain work.

o. *Hemicrania*, caused by congestion ; baths, onct., compr. of A2. El. A. to the corresponding nerves. onct., comp., baths of C5. A II. or A2 II, a b. s. onct. to the heart of A2 onct. or comp. of F2 to the hypoc.

p. *Effusion of the brain*, following on malignant fever. S. Baths of S. C. internally, onct., compr. of S. C5.; baths of C5. comp. of El. B. El. R. "—" El. J. to occ., symp.; comp. to the head of El. R. A. internally with comp. of El. A. to the head.

q. *Rheumatismal Cephalagia of the left side.* S. A. onct., comp., baths of C5 onct. of S. A2. comp. of El. B. El. R. "—" El. J. to occ., symp.; onct. of S5, comp. El. A.

r. *Shooting pains in the head*, El. B. (repeat the applications) and S. internally, onct of S. C. internally and comp. of same. Onct., comp., baths of C5.

s. *Neuralgia of the head* proceeding from cold. El. B. El. R. "—" El. J. baths, onct. to the head of C5 onct. of S; A2, baths of S.

t. *Chronic pains of the head and stomach.* El. R. "—" El. J. to symp., pit of stomach, plex, sol., occ. El. B. to same places, or S. internally with onct. of same to pit of stomach and forehead. Baths of C5, onct. of same to pit of stomach and forehead, comp. of same.

u. *Neuralgia of the head* with stitch in the side. S. a b. s. El. B. to all the nerves of the head, or onct. of S. Baths of S. C5. and A2. El. R. "——" El. J. to occ., symp., plex. sol., onct. of F2 or C5 to the hypoc.

133. Heart-The study of diseases of the heart involves an extended knowledge of pathology. For us, the difl'erent shades of these maladies have very little utility in the administration of the medicines. It is sufiicient to know that the heart is diseased, which can be recognized by the following symptoms: vertigo, palpitation, irregular pulsation of the heart, pain in the left side, shortness of breath, oppression, varicose veins, piles, swelling of the lower extremities, etc. *Treatment:* A II. A2 II. C II. Baths of A2. comp., onct. of A2. Baths of C5. Comp. of C5. or F2. to the hypoc.-Compr. with granules of A2 or A to heart. Moisten the hand with El A. and pass it lightly over the region of the heart. See *Angina pectoris.*

If weight exists in the left side or bilious vomiting add F II alternately with the preceding.

External treatment holds the first rank in heart diseases. Take care that the applications indicated are made on the point the most compromised, for example: the aorta and the carotid arteries. The treatment as described is *certain* in every class of disorder. In some cases 20 gr. of A. or A2. produce a better effect. The greater part of pains proceeding from defective circulation yield to this treatment; these are those which resist the antiscrofolous and red, yellow and white electricities.

Spitting of blood, wounds with hemorrhage, etc., treated the same. (See also *wounds.*)

134. Heart-burn-*Pyrosis*; See *Throat, Stomach.*

135. Hernia-Rupture; El. B., R. or A. to the rupture S. "—" A2. Baths onct., compr., of C5, or S. 20 gr. of C5.

The compresses can be arranged round the circle of the rupture.

136. Herpes-See *Cutaneous diseases.*

137. Hip-Accidental Coxalgia S. and compr. of El. R. or B. to the hip, or 20 gr. of C5. or baths, onct., compr. of S. or C5. or S5.

a. *Spontaneous Coxalgia*; See 137, also 10 gr. of C4. 10 gr. of A2. El. A.

138. Hooping Cough-A III. a b. s. Baths of C5 and onct. A2. to the heart. El. A. to symp., plex. sol., or else the *Pettorali*: or again C III. if there is superabundance of lymph, or C5. III., or baths of El. B.

138. bis. Hoarseness-P. a b. s. C5. a b. s. S. a b. s. gargles of El. R. or B. and with the three first remedies. El. R. "— " El. J. to occ., to great and small hypoglossids. Baths of C5.

139. Humours Cold-S. C C5. C4. Baths of C5 of S. of A2. El. R. "—" El. J. to the symp., occ., plex. sol. El. B.

140. Hydrocele-Tumour of the Testicle. S. C. C5. C4, Baths of S. and A2. Compr. of C5. El. R, "—" El. J. to the symp., occ., plex. sol. El. B.

141. Hydrocephalus-As 140. also onct. of C5. to the whole head.

142. Hypocondria-See *Insanity*.

143. Hysteria-C. II a b. s. S. III a b. s. or for angioitio patients A II a b. s. baths of C5.

144. Hydrophobia-*Canine Madness*; I cannot quote any cure, never having had an occasion to treat a case. But I think that this species of poisoning may be subdued as well as others. I indicate the remedies for those who may happen to have to try them. S. El. R. "—" El. J. to symp., occ., plex. sol. and pit of the stomach.

I

145. Impetigo-Chronic eruption of pustules more or less separated, of which the summit suppurates forming a roughish, yellowish crust scattered or united.

S. II. a b. s. A. a b. s. Baths, compr., onct. to the face of C5. S. onct. of F2. to the hypoc. 20 gr. C5. El. R. "—" El. J. to occ., symp. and all the nerves of the face.

146. Impotence-General prostration. El. R. "—" El. J. to pit of stomach, symp., occ. S. Baths (3 spoonfuls) of El. B. or R, or A. 20 gr. of C5. or 10 gr. of C4.

147. Indigestion-An interrupted digestion is restored by a few granules of S. dry on the tongue, if the symptoms are grave, here give as many as 20; if needed, afterwards the first dilution of scrofoloso in frequent doses. In serious cases, and especially to avoid the consequences, El. R. "—" El. J. to pit of stomach, and plex. sol. or even baths of C5. or S.

148. Influenza, at onset, treatment as in *throat*. Letters c. d.

149. Insanity, Generally treated by S II a. b. s. and baths of C5.

Insanity not arising from any organic defect is *certainly* cured by the *scrofolosi* or (in woman) by the *cancerosi*, and the *angioitici*, or the *vermifughi*.

In women the organs of reproduction, of which C. is the specific, exercise a great influence.

a. *Furious insanity* S. III a. b. s. A2. III a. b. s. baths of C5. El. B. to occ, and symp.

b. Same of 3 years standing, with accesses of fury, see a.

c. Same with loss of speech, see a. also: onct. of C5. and comp. of El. B. to great and little hypoglossids.

d. Woman aged 29 years, cured by small doses (3rd dilution) of C. and El. R. "—" El J to occ., symp., and onct. of C5. to back of neck.

e. Same after confinement. C III a. b. s. El. R. "—" El. J. to occ., symp. Baths of C5, onct. of same to sacred nerves, applications of El. B. to same nerves.

f. *Melancholy:* (Woman aged 24.) cured. See e.

g. *Melancholy:* (Woman aged 57.) S II. a b. s. El. R. "—" El. J. to pit of stomach, occ. compr. of C5. or El. B. to back of neck.

h. *Hypocondria*: S II. a b. s. and F II a b. s. onct. of F2. to the hypoc. and baths of C5. El. R. "—" El. J. to plex. sol., symp. compr. of El. B. to the hypoc.

i. *Nymphomania:* C III a b. s. Baths of C5. comp. C5. or El, B to the sacred nerves.

j. *Paroxysms of fury:* (Man aged 35 years) S II Baths of C5. El. B. to occ., symp.

k. *Idiocy with deafness.* See i.

l. *Imbecility* (woman) C. Baths of C5. compr. of El. B. to sacred nerves. El. R. El. J. to occ., symp., plex. sol. and all the nerves of the head.

m. *Monomania:* see a; but for woman give C. instead of S.

n. *General weakness* of mind and body. See a.

Numerous cures of insanity, hypochondria, monomania have been made at all ages and in both sexes. The cure of the insane! This is really a discovery of the greatest importance.

150. Itch-S II. C II. A2 II. a b. s. Baths of C5. or S. El. R. "—" El. J. to occ., symp., plex. sol. Onct of F2. or C5 to the hypoc. Baths of El. B. or of A2.

151. Itching-See 150.

152. Intermittent (of pains and fevers). F II. a b. s. onct. of F2. or C5. to the hypoc. El. R. "—" El. J. to symp., occ., plex. sol. Baths of C5. or S.

153. Intoxication-10 grains of S. at once dry on the tongue.

a. *Habitual intoxication* and consequences. S II. a b. s. S. A2 II. a b. s. Compr. of F2. to the hypoc. compr. A. to the heart. El. B. to symp. plex. sol. Baths, onct. (to the hypoc.) of C5. El. R. "—" El. J. to occ., symp. 20 gr. of C5.

J

154. Jaundice-F. II. a b. s. onct. of F2. to the hypoc. Baths of C5. El. A. to symp., plex. sol. El. R. "—" El. J. to occ., symp. El. B.

K

155. King's evil-See *scrofula.*

156. Knee-White swelling of-Internal treatment as n° 130. A. externally: onct., baths, compr. of C5., S. or S5., but especially C. internally and externally El. R. "—" El. J. to the corresponding nerves, also El. B.

a. *If painful:* El. V. onct., compr. of C5, of El. B. or El. A.

b. *Periodical Rhemnatism* of: F II. onct. of F2 to the hypoc. In general treat as gout. See *Gout.*

L

157. Legs-Oedema, swelling of) A II. a b s. A 2 II. a b. s. C II. a. b. s. Baths of C5., baths, onct., compr. A2. El. of A. to occ., symp. onct. of F2 to hypoc.

a. *Varicose ulceration:* See *ulcers*, also compr. of El. A.

b. *Varicose ulceration* complicated with scrofula. See *ulcers.* C. C5, A, or A2.

158. Lepra-See *glands.*

Syphilitic ulcerations: Ven. a b. s. and compr. For other treatment refer to glands.

Lepra complicated with epilepsy: C II. a b. s. for other treatment See *glands.*

158. bis. Lethargy-Employ the antiscrofulous or antiangioitics, according to the case, and application of an appropriate electricity to the back of the neck, eyes and symp.

159. Leucorrhea-See *Womb.*

160. Lightening (effects of)-10 grains at once dry on the tongue. .El. R. "—" El. J. to occ., plex. sol., temples, and all the nerves of the head. Compr. El. B. to the head.

161. Lips (hard swelling of)-C. II. a b. s. compr. of C. of El. B. Baths, onct., compr. of C5. 20 gr. of C5.

162. Liver and spleen-Two joint viscera.

Liver diseases may be recognized by the following symptoms: Yellow complexion, urine dense, yellow or reddish; alvine evacuations, greyish or clay color. Pain in right hypochondre; pain at the bottom of the stomach extending to the spine, and ascending to the right shoulder; heaviness of the right side, sometimes bilious vomiting, etc.

Treatment: F. II. a b. s. To the hypoc. employ onct. compr. of F2. C5 El. B. Baths of C5. El. R. "—-" El. J. to symp, plex. sol., occ. If at same time there is affection of the heart alternate A2 II. with F. and apply onct. to the heart with A2. replace El. B. with El. A.

a. *Hepatitis:* Inflammation of the liver F II. a b. s. onct. of C5. and F2. to the hypoc. Compr. baths of C5. also El. R. and J. to plex. sol., symp., bottom of stomach. El. B. to part affected.

b. *Gastrohepatitis:* Inflammation of liver and stomach, F II. a b. s. S II a b. s. onct. of F2. to the hypoc. Baths, compr. of C5. S. El. R. "—" El. J. to pit of stomach, baths of El. B.

c. An affection of the liver, existing 14 years, was cured in ten days by onct. of F2. to the hypoc.

d. *Congestion of liver* complicated with dropsy F II a b. s. comp. of F. to the hypoc. baths of C5 El. B. "—" El. J. to plex sol., symp. comp. of El. B. to the parts, and plex. sol.

e. *Tumour of the liver:* See d. also El. R. "—" El. J. to liver and spleen.

163. Loins-Diseases of the loins.

S. C. C5. A2. Onct., compr. of C5. S. onct. of A2. to the parts. Baths of C5. S. Baths or compr. of El. B. El. R. "—" El. J. to loins and sacred nerves.

a. *Nephritis:* See under this title also *Bladder.*

b. *Consumption* of the: A II. A2 II. a b. s. onct. of A2 to the loins. Baths. of C5. onct. of S. or C5. to loins. Baths, compr. of El. B. El. R. "—" El. J. to the loins.

164. Lockjaw-S. a b. s. El. R. "—" El. J. to the nerves of the jaw, occ., symp. onct. of C5, or S. compr. of El. B. Also El. J. to occ., master nerve, symp. baths of C5. Onct. of C5.

165. Lumbago-Consequent on cold. S. a b. 5. Baths, onct., compr. of C5 or S. compr. of El. B. or El. ' R. "—" El. J. to symp., occ., and sides of the spine.

a. *Accompanied with fever:* F II a b. s., as 165.

b. *Caused by worms:* Ver. a b. s. also 165.

166. Lungs-Nervous cough. S II. C5 II. B2 II. a b. s.

a. *Tuberculous cough*-P II. P2 II. C5 II. S II. a b. s. Onct., compr. to the chest of C5 of S. Bath of C5. S. El. B. El. R. "—" El. J. to occ., symp., plex. sol. Onct. of C4. to the chest.

b. *Congestive cough*, with spitting of blood ; as above, but alternate with A II. or A2 II. the pectorals, and use compr. and onct. of A2 to the chest and heart; baths of A2.

c. *Simple or chronic cough* consequent on cold-P. P2 II. C II. a b. s. Gargles of El. B.

d. *Cough arising from worms*-Ver. II. Ver.2 II. a b. s. See c.

e. *Cough with hectic symptoms*-following on pneumonia and pleurisy, especially in scrofulous patients. C II. a b. s. El. B. and El. J. to symp. See c.

f. *Chronic congestion of the lungs*-P. C5. or P2 II. a b. s.

g. *Acute or Chronic Catarrh*-P II. P2. A2. a b. s.

h. *Chronic Bronchitis with Asthma*-P2 II. P2. P3 II. S II. S5 II. a b. s. Either employed singly or alternately.

i. *Hoarseness*-See h. Gargle of El. B. or R. or A. *N.B.*-C is specific for tubercles at the onset especially.

j. *Influenza*-sorts of acute bronchitis; gargle of El R. stops the malady instantly at its commencement; when the disease is declared. See c. and add alternate gargles of El. R., B. and A.

k. *Dropsy of the chest*, with difficulty of breathing. S II. C II. P II. a b. s. El. R. "—" El. B. to the back of the neck; plex. sol., symp. A.

l. *Inflammation of the lungs*. See g. h.

m. *Pleurisy with fever*. F II. S II. P II. A II. a b. s. El. B. to occ. plex. sol., symp. Onct. of C5 the chest ; Baths of C5.

n. *Pleurodinia* (pains or stitches in the side) disappear at the onset by El. B to the part affected.

o. *Inflammation* of the lungs following on Measles. S II. a b. s. generally sufficient, or else C II. a b. s. or 20 gr. C5.

p. *Phthisis*, with green expectoration, and inflammation of the lungs P II. C II. C5. a b. s. Onct. (to the chest) and baths of C5. El. B. to 0cc., symp., plex. sol S2. S. a b. s.

q. *Tubercular Phthisis*. See q. also F. II a b. s. Onct. of F2 to the hypoc.

r. *Phthisis*, with complications of the larynx. See q. also P2. II. P3. II, a b s.

s. *Oedema* (soft swelling) C II. a b. s. 20 gr. of C5. C2. II. a b. s. Baths of C5. and A2.

t. *Chronic disorganization of the lung*. C II. C5. a b. s. Onct. of F2. to the hypoc. F II. a. b. s. El. B. to plex. sol., symp.. Onct. to the hypoc. of C5.

The cures of phthisis obtained by means of C. P. P2. and baths of C5. are innumerable.

167. Lymph-It is known that the system of circulation comprises: the arteries; which carry the blood from the heart, throughout the whole body, the veins, which bring the blood from all parts of the body to the heart, and the lymphatic vessels, existing in every portion of frame, forming numerous ganglions by their union. The lymphatics empty into the veins a liquid drawn from nearly all parts of the organism and named *lymph*. Lymph is clear, transparent, a little yellowish or greenish, saline, and has a decided alkaline reaction. Its composition contains albumen, fibrine, fat, salts, all dissolved in water. It is remarkable that the quantity of fibrine goes on increasing, from the source of the lymphatic system to its discharge into the veins; it is in this respect that the blood may be considered a continuation of the lymph, it will, also, be understood that alterations of the lymph produce the same in the blood and *vice-versa*. Diseases of the lymph, by far the most numerous, demand especially the antiscrofulous and anticancerous.

Soft, flabby flesh, diaphanous skin and watery blood point out the lymphatic temperament.

168. Marasmus (Wasting away)-S. a b. s. El. R. "—" El. J. to occ. symp. plex. sol. onct. of C2. to the whole of the head. El. B. to the head.

169. Marasmus general-With ancylosis (enlargement of the joints). *See* 168. Also baths of C5 S. or A2.

170. Masturbation-S. II. a b. s.-Involuntary nocturnal emissions. 20 gr. of C5 El. R. "—" El. J. to occ. symp. plex. sol. comp. El. B. to occ. Baths of S5.

171. Measles-See *fevers*.

172. Melancholy (Compare Insanity)-S. II a b. s. If proceeding from the womb. C. II a b. s.

173. Meloena-Vomiting of black blood, commonly called black Bile. Flow of dark coloured blood from the digestive organs, and voided either by the mouth or the anus. A. II. or A2 II. a b. s. comp. to the heart of A. El. A. to symp. plex. sol. baths, onct. or compr. of A2. Baths of C5. El. R. "—" El. J. to occ. to sides of seventh vertebra (base of the neck) El. B. Compare *Vomiting.*

174. Mercurial salivation-with special apthes in the mouth. S. a b. s. or C. a b. s. or C5. a b. s. or 20 gr. C5. or baths of C5. El. R. "—" El. J. to occ. symp. hypoglosses sub orbitals.

175. Menses-Menhorrhagia, haemorrage of the womb. A. II a b. s. and compr. A. or A2 to the heart. Baths of El. A. C. A2 and comp. to the heart of same. El. A. to the sacrum. In same case, granules of angioitics dry give the best results.

a. *Amenorrhoea,* (suppression of the menses) *See* 175. In particular cases good effects are obtained by S. "—" C. "—" A.

b. *Profuse menstruation. See 175.* It is to be remembered, that: *angioitics in ordinary doses bring back the menses, whereas, at the second dilution, they moderate and even arrest the flow.*

c. *Dysmenorrhoea,* abnormal and painful menstruation. S. "—" C. "—" A2.

d. Same with swelling of the nose, *see 175*, Comp. onct. of A2. or C5. to the nose. El. A. to the base of nose. Baths of C5.

e. *Same* chronic, *see* c. El. A. to sacred nerves. Baths of A2. onct. of A'. to sacred nerves and the heart.

f. *Sudden suppression of the menses* (caused by cold water) with headache. Compr. El. B, to occ. symp. to super orbitals and temples. S. C5. Baths of C5.

g. *Suppression with chlorosis. See 175.*

h. *Permature cessation. See 175.*

176. Mesenteric disease-*See abdomen* letter c.

177. Milk, Flow of, when not suckling (galactorrhoea) C II "—" A2 II a b. s. baths of C5. El. R. and El. J. to occ., symp., plex. sol. Baths of El. B. or of S. S3. 20 gr. C5.

178. Milk fever-Suppression of Milk. C. II C5 II. a b. s. compr. to the breast of El. B. El. R. "—" El. J. to symp., plex. sol , occ.

179. Mouth-Stomaeh complaints; fetidity of the mouth. Gargles of El. R. or El. B. or of S. C. El. R. "— " El. J. to pit of the stomach, and plex. sol. Baths, onct. of C5. to the parts, or baths, onct of S. or baths of A2.

a. Increase the fetidity, during menstruation; as 179 also A2. internally.

b. Impossibility of opening the mouth. El. R. to occ., symp. to the masseter muscles. Onct. and baths of C5. or onct. of S. A single application of electricity has often been suflicient.

N

180. Nausea-Also of pregnancy. C. S. C5 a b. s. Baths of C5. 10 gr. of C4.

181. Nephritis-Inflammation of the kidneys. S. A2. a b. s. Baths, onct. (to the loins) compr. of C5. or S5 or S. onct of F2 to the hypoc. or C5. Baths of El. B. El. R. "—" EL J. to occ., symp. and the length of the spine.

182. Nerves-(diseases of), as 181.

a. *Nervous agitation:* S II. or A II. a b. s. light applications of El. B. to occ., symp., plex. sol. For angioitic patients, compr. to the heart of A2. see also 183.

b. *Alteration of the nerves from abuse of quinine.* S. a b. s. Baths of C5 El. R. "—" El. J. to symp., or bath of El. B.

183. Nervous agitation-In general S III. a b.s. Baths of C5. El. B. to symp. Baths of S. Onct C5. to the whole of the head.

184. Nervous contractions of the whole body. Ordinarily removed by El. R. to symp., occ., plex. sol. Baths of G5. which may be alternated with baths of El. B.

185. Neuralgia-See also *Pains.*

a. *Accidental nervous pains;* cured instantly by comp. El. B. or applications of El. R. or J. or. when the individual is angioitic, A.

If these means do not succeed, try compr., onct.; baths of C5. S. or A2. or S5. S. a b. s.

b. *Congestive neuralgia.* A. or A2 a b. s comp., onct, baths of A2. baths of El. A. of El. B.

c. *Syphilitic neuralgia.* Ven II. a b. s. Baths (100 globules) of Ven. Baths, onct., comp. of C5. S. S5. El. B. in compresses to painful parts. El. R. "—" El. J. Onct of F2. or C5. to the hypoc.

d. *General neuralgia.* See c. also baths, onct. compr. of A2.

e. *Neuralgia of the head with rheumatism of the arm.* See c.

f. *Dental neuralgia.* See c. also gargles of S. A2. C. and C5. and S5.

186. Nocturnal pollutions-S. II. A2. b. s. C5. baths, onct. (to sacred nerves) of C5. of S. El. B. to sacred nerves, pubis and perineum. El. R. El. J. to occ., symp., plex. sol., and sacred nerves. Onct. of F2. to the hypoc.

187. Nodes-Bony tumours developed on the surface of a bone, generally consequent on syphilitic or scrofulous diseases, accompanied by violent pains. S. C. A. C5. C4. Onct., compr., baths of C5, S. or S5.

Compr. of Ven. 20 gr. of C5. or S5. or S. or C4.

Compr. of El. B. or El. R.

a. *Syphilitic Nodes.* Ven. internally and in compresses. Treat as above.

b. *Periostitis*; scrofulous or not. See 187. Also onct. of S. or A2.

c. *Spina Ventosa*. Dilation of the tissues of the bones, as if they were blown out.-Sharp and severe pains; treat with *cancerosi* and as 187.

d. *Treatment of ricketty children*. S. S2. or *nuovo*, C. a b. s. S5. A2. Baths onct. compr. of C5. or S. or S5. Baths of A2. or El. B. or El. A. El. R. "—" El. J. to occ., symp., plex. sol. and all the nerves corresponding to the affected parts. Baths of El. R. or El. V.

e. *Chronic Node* On the right leg; See d. persist in onct. of S. of A2. Compr. El. V.

f. *Same* on the lower jaw, with fever. See e. Also F II. a b. s.

g. *Same* with retraction of the jaw. See e., but especially use C. internally and in compresses.

h. *Spina Ventosa* in the foot with several lemon color wounds. Amputation proposed ; but the foot was cured in following treatment indicated letter e; persisting especially with C. and El. V. The decayed bone will be seen to come away in pieces.

i. *Softening of the bones*. (Rickets) See d. persist in baths of C5. and El. V.

188. Nose-Ozoena, (ulcer of the nose). S. a b. s. C. a b. s. A2. a b. s. C5. a b. s. Inhalation of these remedies, and onct. to the base of the nose of C5. El. R. "—" El. J. to the occ., symp., eyes and base of the nose. Baths of C5. El. B. S. A2. and S5. The cure is certain.

a. *Suppuration* of the nose. *See* 188.

b. *Swelling* of the nose. *See* 188.

c. *Ulceration* of the nose. *See* 188, but C. C5. A2. are preferable.

d. *Polypus* of the nose. *See* c.

e. *Cancerous vegetation* at the base of the nose. *See* e. Compr. El. B. to base of nose.

f. *Epistaxes*: bleeding from the nose. A. or A2. or C5. a b. s. Inhalation of the same medicines. El. A. to base of the nose, occ., symp., to forehead, or baths, onct., compr. of A2. Compr. to the heart of A2.

The doses, relatively too strong, increase the affection.

g. *Scrofulous Ozoena* from infancy; *See* 188. Also C5. internally; inhalations, onctions externally.

h. *Dry Polypus* of the nose, with gangrene. *See* g.

189. Nose (Bleeding of)-See *Epistaxis.*

190. Nymphomania-C II. a b. s. C5. a b. s. or 20 gr. C5. or C4. Baths of C5. Onct., compr. to pubis and sacred nerves of C5. El. B. to symp., plex. sol., back of the neck and sacred nerves. Baths of S5.

O

191. Obesity-S. C. or C4. or C5. a b. s. Baths, onct. (to the pit of the stomach) of C5. El. B. (to the same place) El. R. "—" El. J. to occ. symp. plex. sol. Baths of S. A2. onct. to the hypoc. of F2. or C5.

192. Obesity morbid-(Unhealthy stoutness) S. or Ven. or A. or A2. or 20 gr. of this last. Baths of C5. or S. or A2. El. R. "—" El. J. to symp occ. plex. sol. Baths of El. B.

P

193. Palate (polypus of)-C. a b. s. Gargle of C. C5. a b. s. Gargle of C5. of A2. of El. B. C4. and El. R. Baths of C5.

194. Paralysis (commencement and threateningof)-Averted by 10 or 12 granules of S. given dry on the tongue, or, else, bathe the head with El. B. or El. R. "—" El. J. to occ., symp. plex. sol. Onct., compr. to the head with C5. or S.

a. *Menace of general Paralysis.* El. R. to symp., plex. sol., but especially to the pit of the stomach.

When there is congestion, A2 II. A II. a b. s. Compr. to the heart with these remedies and baths of A2. El. A. to all the nerves of the head, especially to occ., symp.' and temples. The means should be persevered in until the recovery of the patient. In case of doubt as to the cause, alternate the anti-angioitics with the anti-scrofulous, preferring those which produce favourable effects.

If the patient experiences some unpleasant effects from an erroneous remedy, a few globules of S., dry on the tongue, will promptly remove them. If unsuccessful C. C5. C4. should be employed, but the first especially.

b. *Nervous paralysis without any symptoms of angioitics.*

S. C. C5. A. S5. Baths of the head of El. B. El. R. "—" El. J. to occ., symp., plex. sol. and all the nerves of the head. Baths of El. B. or C5. S. or A2.

c. *Paralysis consequent on a sanguine apoplexy.* A. A2. II. a b. s. compr. to the heart of A. or A2. onct. or comp. to the hypoc. of C5. or F2. Baths of El. A. (2 or 3 tablespoonfuls) C. S. onct. to the entire head of A2.

In some cases El. J. to Occ. has been successful.

d. *Nervous paralysis of the tongue*, S. a b. s. gargle of S. El. B. and C5. onct. comp. of C5. to hypoglossids. El. R. "—" El. J. to little hypogloss, occ. symp. baths of S. and C5.

e. *Congestive paralysis of the tongue.* A II. A2 II. comp. to the heart of A. gargle with A. A2. El. A. onct. of A2. to hypoglos. baths of A2.

f. *Paralysis of half the body.* S. A. onct. or comp. to the hypoc. of C5. Baths of C5, of S. and A2. El. B. to the whole body, or El. A. passed lightly over the head. Comp. to the heart of A. 10 gr. of A2. El. R. "—" El. J. to symp., occ., plex. sol., super orbitals.

g. *Paralysis of one side of the face.* El. R. and El. J. to occ., symp., forehead, sub orbitals, base of nose, and masseter muscle, compr. of El. B.

S. S5 or C5 internally, alternated with A., at same time, onct. to the part affected and the whole head of C5, baths of C5, S5. If these remedies are resisted, use C. A2.

h. *Paralysis of the eyelids.* S. A. onct. baths of C5. onct. of S. and A2. El. B. or El. A. in compresses El. R. "—" El. J. to super and sub orbital, root of nose, symp. plex. sol.

i. *Paralysis of arm or leg. See* f. onct. of C5.

j. *Paralysis of the prostrate gland.* See f. Onct. to sacrum, perineum, pubis of C5. S. El. R. or El. B. in compresses to the same parts.

k. *Paralysis of the bladder. See* J.

l. *General Hemiplegia* consequent on an apoplexy, with varicose veins and varicose ulcers, etc. A. A2. Baths, onct. compr. of A2. Baths of C5, compr. of El. A2 to all the nerves of the head, and along the spine, onct. to the hypoc. of F2 or C5. Baths of C5, El. B. and El. A.

m. *Paralysis of the left side. See* b., also onct. to the part of C5, S., A2.

n. *Paralysis of the genital organs.* S. A. onct. to the parts of C5. S. A2. Baths of the same remedies. El. R. "—" El, J. to sacred nerves, pubis and perineum. Baths of El. B. or El. A.

o. *Paralysis of the legs,* following small pox. *See* 194. Also onction, comp. of C5. A2. El. B. Baths of El. B.

195. Pains, (Neuralgic) etc.-El. R. or El. J. or El. R. "—" El. J. S. A. C5. Baths of C5. and especially onct. of C5. S. and A2. to the part.

a. *Cephalalgia-See* 195 and comp. El. B. to super orbital.

b. *Pains* in the right side. onct. of F2 to the hypoc and F. a b. s. comp. El. B.

c. *Pains* during the night. Ven. a b. s., the rest as 195. Baths of S. C5, A2, S5.

d. *Pains* in the left side. A II. A2. II. a b. s. Baths of C5. comp of A2. to the region of the heart. El. A. to symp.

e. *Pains* at about a third of the sacrum. Ven. II. a b. s. comp. of Ven. or onct. of C5. Baths of the same or of S. Baths of El. B. onct. of S.

f. *Pain* of the skull under the saggittal seam. C. II. a b. s. compr., onct. of C5. and C. baths of C5. or compr. of El. B.

g. *Pain* in the bone of the nose. Ven. II a b. s. Onct. of Ven. of C5. or S. Compr. El. B. Generally, for these kinds of pains, C. II. a b. s. or 10 gr. of C.

h. *Deep seated pains* in the bones, as if they were fractured. S. II a b. s. baths, onct., compr. of S. A2. El. A. to occ., symp. and onct. of C5. to the spot; or bath of C5. Compr. El. B. Bl. R. "—" El. J.

i. *Syphilitic pains*. Ven. II. a b. s. El. V. the rest as above, h.

j. *Pain* in the knee, from white swelling, El. R. and El. J. to corresponding nerves. compr., onct., baths of C5. El. B. or El. A. or C5.

k. *Pain in the arm* from a fall, El. R. "—" El. J. Compr., onct., baths of C5. or S. with S. or A. internally. Compr., onct. (to the arm) and also bath of A2.

l. *Neuralgic pain* of left temple, of 21 years standing, removed by compr. El. B.

m. *Shooting gouty pain* in thumb joint El. V. *See* k.

n. *Spasmodic and rheumatic pain* in foot, existing 10 years cured in a man aged 23; The same, in the hand, of 18 years standing, cured instantly in a man aged 47 years.

o. *Painful sensations* of the whole body. Baths of C5. or 30 gran. of the same; baths of S. or A2. El. R or El. J. to all the nerves.

p. *Uncertain pains* removed in a man aged 39 years. El. R. to occ., symp., plex. sol. *See* o.

q. *Remains of articular pains*: Onct., baths of C5. *See* o.

r. *Pain* in the shoulder, consequent on exertion. The shoulder was replaced by S. and El. R. "—" El. J. also can be employed baths, onct., compr. of S. or C5.- Oompr. El. B. baths of A2.

s. *Pains* left by ancient small-pox. El. R. "—" El. J. or comp. El. R. or onct., baths of C5. or *see* o. Ven. internally can also by tried.

t. *Pains* and helplessness of the arm; El. R. "—" El. J. *See* s.

u. *Pain* in arm, consequence of fall, with affection of liver: as v. cure finished by F. internally.

v. *Shooting pain* in the fold of the anus, with rheumatism. S. onct. (to the part) baths, compr. of C5. or else, baths, onct., compr. of S. or baths of A2. or S5.

The pains, removed by the simple electricity, are innumerable; when one has, once, acquired the habit of using these liquids, it is. merely, a child's game to relieve pain. It is necessary not to forget that the electricities cannot cure without relapse, always, pains proceeding from a profound viciation, which claims jointly an internal treatment.

196. Pemphigus-Eruption of bladders, preceded by general uneasiness (vesicular fever), F. II. a b. s. onct. to the hypoc. of F2. Baths, compr. of C5. of S. and A2. El. R. "—" El. J. to plex. sol., symp., occ. Baths of El. B. Onct. to the hypoc. of C5, S II. a. b. s. 20 gr. C5.

197. Peritonitis-C II. a b. s. compr. C. baths, onct., compr. of C5. onct. to the hypoc. of F2. El. R. "—" El. J. to symp., plex. sol. Compr. El. B. to abdomen See *Abdomen*.

198. Pericarditis-(Compare *Heart*) C III. or A2. III. a b. s. apply onct. to the heart of A, or A2 with 2 gr. of remedy to spoonful of oil. Baths of C5. onct. to the hypoc. of C5. or F2. El A.

199. Perspiration, excessive, with headache. S. El. R. "—" El. J. to occ., symp., plex. sol. Baths of El. B. of C5. S. and A2. onct. to the hypoc. F2. 20 gr. of C5. For suppressed perspiration, the same remedies.

200. Perspiration, excessive and fetid of the feet and arm pits. S. C. C2. C4. A2. a b. s. Baths of C5 S. S5. and El. B. or El. R. "—" El. J. to occ., symp. See also *Feet*.

201. Pimples on the face-See *Face*.

202. Piles in general-See *Hemorrhage*. Alternate S II. with the angioitics.

a. *Bleeding piles*: as above.

b. *Painful piles*, with fissure of the anus. As above, and also baths, onct. , compr. of C5.

203. Poisoning and its consequences-S. or 20 gr. of same. The *Scrofoloso* expels poison. El. R. "—" El. J. to occ.. symp., plex. sol. Baths of S. or A2. or S5.

204. Pregnancy, difficult or painful-C II. or 10 gr. of C5. relieve at once, El. B. to the sacred nerves.

205. Polypi-See *Nose, Womb, Bladder, Pabis*. Persist in C5. internally, and unctions, inhalations, injections of the same.

206. Prolapsus Ani-S. C5. El. R. "—" El. J. to sacred nerves, perineum. Baths, and onct. of C 5. to the part. Baths, compr. S. Injections or clysters of El. B. baths of A2.

a. *Prolapsus Uteri*; as above, but replace S. by C. internally.

207. Prolapsus Uteri-Falling of the womb. C. A2. onct. of C5. to pubis, to sacred nerves, injections of C5. El. R. "—" El. J. to sacred nerves and pubis. Injections of El. B. Baths of S. or C5.

208. Proud flesh-Morbid development of the sanguine vessels. A II. A2 II. C. alternated, compr., onct., baths of S5. or baths, onct., compr. of C5. Baths, onct., compr. of A2. compr. of El. B. El. R. "—" El. J. to the loins. Compr. El. A. or A2 to the heart.

209. Pruritus-Intolerable itching, with eruptions of little hard pimples, like millet grains. S. A. Baths of C5. S. A2. El. R. "—" El. J. to symp., occ., plex. sol.

Of the whole body: as above, and frequent baths of C5.

210. Pustule malignant-See *Carbuncle*.

211. Pubis-See *Womb. Generation* (organs of). Eruption of the polypi on pubis. See *Lepra*. Also Ven. C a b. s. or S. or 20 gr. C5.

212. Prostration of strength-Sometimes a single application of El. R. to the pit of the stomach re-establishes the forces. If the prostration continues, apply electricity to all the nerves of the head, and sides of the spine.

In general S. or 20 gr. C5. El. R. and El. J. to the above mentioned nerves comp. of El. B. or El. A.

Q

213. Quinsy-C II. if the tonsils are not attacked, S. II. and gargles of C. or C5. compr., onct. of C5. to the throat, or bath of C5. El. R. "—" El. J. to back of neck; onct. of S.

R

214. Rectum (Fall of)-C II. a b. s. Baths onct., compr. of C5., or S., or S5. Compr. El. B. Injections of C5. El. B. "—" El. J. the length of the spine and perineum. Also C. Compr. C. and S. Baths of El. B. or R. El. R. "—" El. J. to symp. and sacred nerves. Baths, onct., and compr. of C5.

215. Rectum (loss of blood from)-In a particular case, a cure was made of this disease of 10 years standing, by S a b. s. and compr. to the hypoc of F2. In general S. A II. A2 II. C. a b. s. El. R. "—" El. J. to pit of stomach, plex. sol. Baths of C5. onct. to the hypoc. of C5. baths of A2.

216. Rickets-Softening and deformation of the bones. C. S. A2. or 20 gr. C5. Baths, onct., compr. S. A2. or C5. Baths of El. B. El. R El. A. Onct. to the hypoc. of F2. El. R. El. J. to all the nerves. Onct. to the whole of the head of C5. Baths El. V.

217. Rigidity of the muscles as *216*.

218. Rheumatism-Compare also *Pains*.

Rheumatism generally yields to the application of El. R. and El J. alternated. If it resists these means (by which it is always necessary to begin) or returns repeatedly, the following remedies must be given. S. onct., baths, comp. of S. or baths, compr., onct. of S5. or baths of El. A. and of A2.

a. *Chronic Rheumatism, with nephritis.* See *Nephritis* and *218*, also add El. V.

b. *Articular rhemnatism*: El V. in compr. or as cupping. Baths of S. C5. S5. A2. and as *218*.

Good results have been obtained by the other electricities and onct. of C5. S. C4 . and F2.

c. *Rheumatism of the arm*, very frequently relieved by El. R. to the nerves of the arm.

d. *Chronic rheumatism* with inflammation of the loins, cured by El. R. only, in general as *218*.

e. *Rheumatism* which lasted 50 days and prevented any movement, was cured in one day by S.

Same in both hands cured by S. alone, internally and externally.

Same of 10 years standing, in one hand, with very violent paroxysms, cured by S. internally and externally.

Same but acute, confining the patient to his bed. S. alone internally and externally.

f. *Intercostal Rheumatism.* with suppression of the menses. Cured by A2. alone, internally and externally.

g. Man aged 23 years, attacked by rheumatism in the knees and feet, carried on a man's back to my audience, went away cured by a simple application of El. R.

h. *Chronic Rheumatismal state* with acute crisis by intervals. See *218*.

To S., taken at first dilution, can also be added, according to the case, A2 II.

S

219. St. Vitus's Dance-Chorea S. II a b. s. C5. a b. s. El. R. "— " El. J. to occ. symp., plex sol. Onct of A2. to the heart. Baths of C5 onct. to the whole head of C5. baths of S. or S5.

220. Salivation, and frequent need to expectorate. (Sialorrhoea) For children. Ver. II. a b. s. onct. compr. of C5. to the hypoc. For adults S. gargles of El. B.

The sialorrhoea (continual flow of saliva night and day) of authors can, only, be an affection symptomatic of hysteria, gout, hypochondria, etc.

In these cases the remedy must be directed to the main disease.

221. Scald head of infants-Give the nurse S. or 20 gr. C5. Apply onct. of C5. to the affected part.

Tinea capitis, Tinea farosa, etc., etc., difi'erent eruptions having their seat especially on the scalp, but which, also, appear on other parts of the body, having the form, sometimes, of an agglomeration of pustules, discharging a thick, offensive humour, sometimes furfuraceous scabs, or excavated or raised tubercles, etc.

C. C4. C5. S. S2. S5. a b. s. or A. baths of C5. of S. A2. or S5. Onct. of S5. S. and C5. to the afl'ected parts. Compr. El. B. or El. A. or El. R. El. R. "—" El. J. to occ. and symp. Compr. C4 and S2.

222. Scarlatina-See *Fevers.*

223. Sciatica-Applications of electricities, alone, are frequently sufficient El. R. "—" El. J. to the sacred nerves, to the three points where the nerve is nearest the skin. (See diagram, at end of the book) S II. a b. s. C II. a b. s. or onct., compr., baths of C5. of S S5. or 20 gr. C5. or compr. El. B.

These means are not, always, sufficient in the case of sanguine temperament. For such: El. A. Baths, onct., compr. A2. onct. to the hypoc. either of C5. or F2. Baths of C5. Compr. to the heart with granules of A. or A2. Compr. El. B. onct. of S.

a. *Sciatica*, with biliary calculus, (which was the principal cause of the pain) treated and cured by F2. II. a b. s. onct. of F2 to the hypoc. Onct., of C5. to the hypoc. El. R. El. J. to sciatic nerve, plex. sol., symp., loins; compr., to same parts, of El. B. baths of C5 and S5.

b. *Very painful Sciatica*; cured by S. internally and externally.

c. *Contraction of the sciatic* nerve, cured by S. internally and externally, and compr. of El. R. to the nerve.

d. *Chronic sciatica*, with sharp crisis, preventing the patient from walking, cured by preceeding treatment.

224. Scirrhus-See *Cancer, Womb*, and *Stomach.*

225. Scrotum-See *Testicles, Tumors.*

226. Scrofula-Constitutional disease, constituted by many affections, of which the principal characters are, the tendency to a chronic state, to ulceration, to suppuration, and a deposit of tuberculous matter, principally in the lymphatic ganglions, situated under the lower jaw, and along the neck, the groins, under the armpits, the poplitic hollow, etc.

General treatment. S. a b. s. C. C5. a b. s. 20 gr. of C5. Baths of S. A2. C5. S5. of El. B. El. R. or El. V. Application, of electricity to symp., occ., plex. sol. Onct. or compr. to the hypoc. of F2 or C5.

Science (*Lebert, Traite partique des maladies scrofuleuses et tuberculeuses, Paris, 1849*) recognizes the scrofulous origin of the following diseases, which, in eifect, yield to all the antiscrofulous or their congeners, the anticancerous, namely: the glands in general, afi'ections and eruptions of the skin, such as superficial cutaneous affections, pimples, and tinea, *Lupus vorax* of the face and vulva, cold tumours, abcesses, ulcers, fistulas the great portion of opthalmias, otorrhoea, many alterations of the cartilage and the bones, arthritis, contractions, ancylosis, periostitis, ostetis, necrosis, carries in general, tubercles of the lungs, the stomach, bowels, and uro-urinary organs. Science, also recognizes for the scrofula diagnosis the following symptoms, namely: cough, expectoration, hoemoptisis, pains in the chest, dysuria, fever accompanied by perspirations, laryngitis, tracheitis, pneumonia, pleurisy, pulmonary perforation, chronic gastritis, enteritis, peritonitis, meningitis, tubercular orchitis; afl'ections of the menses, aphthae, etc.

All these maladies are cured by the antiscrofulous, supported, if necessary, by the anticancerous. But, according to us, maladies, cured by the same remedy, have a common origin. Thus our results confirm that which science has declared.

But, there are a great number of diseases, not comprised in the preceding list (here it is sufficient to call to mind that nine tenths of complaints call for the antiscrofulous. See n° 14), which equally yield to the antiscrofulous. Hence, again, it results, in our opinion, that the frame of man is impregnated with scrofulous or psoric principles, which are the source of the greatest part of our infirmitics.

For the treatment of scrofulous diseases, refer to each one, in the catalogue.

227. Sea sickness-Granules of S. dry, each time that the malady commences. S. II. a b. s.

228. Skin. *Ulcerations of the skin.* C. S. A, a b. s. comp. of these remedies, of El. B. or A, or El. R. or C5, or S. El. R. "—" El. J. to occ. symp. plex. sol. Baths, onct. comp. of A2. compr. to the hypoc. of F2. The ulcerations, unless they are supported by some serious viciation, heal easily, even those of cancer, at the end of its cure.

a. *Impetigo, scaly herpes*, as 228, also comp. C. and sometimes V. alone.

b. *Intertrigo*, redness and irritation of the skin, as 228; persist with compr. of El. B. when it is caused by chafing of clothing or by the urine in infants.

c. *Tinea*, as 228; compr. of C5, of S, of A2, see also *Scald head*.

229. Skin (spots on) wine coloured. A, A2 a b. s. compr. onct, baths A2. compr. and baths of El. A, onct. to the heart of A. Baths, onct. of C5. to the part.

Liver Spots on the skin-F II. Onct. to the hypoc. of F2, or C5, or S. Baths of C5. El. C. to the hypoc. Baths of El. R.

Copper coloured patches on skin. See *Syphilis*.

Specks in the cornea-See *Eyes*.

230. Sleeplessness-El. R. and El. J. to symp. occ. plex. sol. and all the nerves of the head. S. a b. s. 20 gr. of C5. or onct. to the hypoc. of F2, or C5. Baths of C5 or S. onct. to the head of S. Bathe the head lightly with El. B.

231. Small Pox-See *Fevers*.

232. Smell (loss or perversion of the sense of)-EI. R. "—" El. J. to base of the nose: onct. comp. of C5, S, A2 to base of the nose. Baths of C5. Inhalations of S, or S a b. s.

233. Sobbing With flatulence-S II a b. s. C5 II a b. s. El. R. to symp. and bottom of the stomach. Little compresses of El. B. to the stomach. Sometimes removed by a simple touch of El. R. to the occiput.

234. Somnambulism in woman-C II C5. II a b. s. Baths of C5, onct. to the hypoc. of the same. El. B. to occ. or baths of the same. .In man. S. S5 and other remedies as above.

a. *Sudden starts, trembling,* etc. See *234.*

235. Spasms, proceeding from worms-Ver. a b. s. Ver. 2 II. a b. s. S. a b. s. Baths with El. B. or C5. S. or A2.

236. Speech (difficulty of)-Generally and immediately restored by applications of El. R. "—" El. to the hypoglossids and occ., symp. See *237* and Stammering.

237. Speech (loss of)-S. a b. s. C. a b. s. A2. a b. s. C5. a b. s. C4 a b. s. Baths, onct., (to the whole head) of C5. or S. El. B. to entire head. El. R. "—" El. J. to occ., symp., plex. sol., hypogl. onct. to the hypoc of F2. and C5.

238. Spermatorrhoea-Compare *Urine, organs of generation.* Involuntary loss of semen. S. II, C. II, a b. s. Baths of C5. S. El. B. El. R. "—" El. J. to perineum and sacred nerves. Injections, in serious cases, of S. A. and C5. onct. or compr. of F2. to the hypoc.

239. Spine-Acute or chronic inflammation of the spinal marrow. S II. a b. s. C II. a b. s. C2. A. a b. s. But, specially, baths and onct. (to the whole head) of C5. or baths of A2. or S., never the electricities before convalescence. At this time, apply comp. of El. B. the length of the spine. El. R. "—" El. J. to occ., symp., temples, and sides of the seventh vertebra and the entire back bone.

a. *Displacement of vertebra*; see *239*, but employ the electricities at the onset.

b. *Curvature of the spine*; see *a.*

c. *Humpback*; see *a.*

240. Spinal marrow, affections of-C2 II a b. s. S II a b. s. A2 II. a b. s. baths, onct., comp. of C5 of S. S5, onct. to the hypoc. of F2: 20 gr. of C5 or S5 or C4 or S2 or *nuovo.* Baths of El. B. When the pain recommences, El. R. "— " El. J. to symp., plex. sol. onct. of C5 to the hypoc.; see also *239.*

241. Spine Ventosa-See *Nodes.*

242. Spleen-The affections of this organ produce the most strange phenomena. Inflammation of the spleen, F II a b. s., comp and onct. to the hypoc. of F2 C5, Baths of C5 10 gr. of C5. Baths of El. B. El. R. "—" El. J. to symp., plex. sol. onct. of S. A2 to the hypoc. See *Liver.*

243. Spitting of blood-Hoemoptisis. A. A2. C5 Baths of C5, onct. of F2 to the hypoc. Baths onct., comp. (to heart) of A2. ELA. to symp. occ., or C II.

244. Sprains-S. a b. s. or 20 gr. of S. C5. a b. s. or 20 gr. of C5. bath of C5. S. A2. or El. B. El. R. "—" El. J. to all the nerves of the part; and to occ., symp., plex. sol. onct. of S. or S5.

245. Stammering, stuttering-Gargles with El. R. or El. B. S. El. R. and El. J. to the little hypoglossids. Baths of C5. Onct. of same to hypogl. Onct. also of A2.

Congenital. as 245. Sometimes has been removed by a single application of electricity.

246. Staphyloma-See *eyes.*

247. Stiff neck, crick in the neck-When with fever. F. and onct. to the hypoc. of F2. or C5. Without, or after fever has subsided, S. and onct. of S. to the part and A2. El. B. in compr. Baths of C5. onct. of S5. El. R. to back of neck or El. R. "—" El. J. to same part.

248. Stings of Insects-C. a b. s. compr. of C. of El. R. El. B. and El. A. onct., compr. of C5. or S.

249. Stomach (Weakness of)-El. R. "—" El. J. to plex. sol., symp. S. a b. s. S5. a b. s. or 20 gr. of this. El. B. to pit of stomach.

a. *Gastritis, Gastralgia.* El. R. "—" El. J. to pit of stomach, onct. of F2. or C5 to hypoc. See also 249.

b. *Pyrosis.* Heartburn; S. A. compr., or baths of C5. or C5. a b. s. El. R. "—" El. J. to occ., symp. compr. of El. B. or El. A.

c. *Indigestion* etc. S. or 20 gr. of S. or S5. or onct. to the hypoc. of F2. El. R. "—" El. J. to symp., plex. sol. Baths of C5, or El. B. for severe derangement of the stomach.

d. *Ulceration of stomach.* See *Cancer.* N.B. Ulcerations produce vomiting of pus and blood; scirrhus throws up a coffee colored discharge.

e. *Nervous Gastritis.* F. II. compr. to the hypoc. of F. or F2. El. B. to symp, plex. sol. Baths of C5. or A2. onct. to hypoc. of C5. or A2.

f. *Convulsions of the bottom of the stomach.* See *e.* also S. II. a b. s. compr. or onct to the hypoc. of F2. or C5. onct. of S. to the part.

g. *Dilation of the stomach.* S. C5. S5. onct. to the hypoc. of F2. or C5. El. B. to symp., plex. sol. El. R. "—" El. J. onct., compr. of C5. to bottom of stomach (see diagram) Baths of C5. or El. B.

h. *Tumour* at the upper (cardiac) orifice of the stomach, C. II. a b. s., C5. II. a b. s. El. R. "—" El. J. to plex. sol. symp. compr. to same parts of El. B. or onct. or baths of C5. Baths of S. or S5. onct. to the hypoc. of F2.

i. *Gastralgia*, accompanied with periodical vomiting, cramps (remains of ancient syphilis) F Ven. onct. to the hypoc. of F2. or C5. El. A. Compr. to hypoc. of C5. or El. R. "—" El. J. to symp., plex. sol. or El. B. to aforesaid parts. Baths of C5. S. and S5.

j. *Gastralgia, after a meal, with violent pain.* See *i*, also onct. of C5 to the painful part.

The cures of stomach complaints, of all descriptions, cannot be counted.

250. Stomatitis-See *Mouth, Stomach.*

251. Stone-See *Bladder.* S. has an elective action on stone.

252. Stratismus, squinting-See *Eyes.*

253. Strangury-See *Bladder*.

254. Strictures, in general. whatever they may be.-See *Loins*, using especially onct. and comp. of C5 and A2.

255. Stupor, produced by the abuse of quinine. El. R. "—" El. J. to occ., symp., plex. sol. and the entire head. S. Baths of C5, or S, or A2, El. B.

256. Stupidity-If proceeding from humours: S. a b. s. El. R. "—" El. J. to occ., symp., plex. sol., baths of El. B. of C5, of S. onct. to the head of S. C5. A2.

If proceeding from disease of the liver: F II a b. s. onct. to the hypoc. of F2, C5, rest as above. If caused by a fall: insist on the baths above mentioned. When caused by fright: A II, A2 II a b. s. comp. onct. to whole of the head A2. baths of the same or El. A.

There are cases of cure by some applications of El. R to occ., symp., plex sol.

251. Suicide (disposition to)-S. II a b. s. baths of C5, of El. B., El. R "—" El. J. to occ., symp., plex. sol. 20 gr. C5. Baths of S.

258. Sunstroke-El. R. "—" El. J. occ., symp., super and sub orbit., forehead. Onct. (to the head), baths of C5. compr. El. B.

Also, El. R. to back of neck, occ., symp., sides of the seventh vertebra, and all the nerves of the head. Onct. or comp. to the head of C5, S., a b. s. 20 gr. of C5. Baths of C5, or S.

259. Swelling of the face (cold in the face)-S. Comp. onct. Baths of C5. El. R. "—" El. J. to sub. orbit. masseter, occ. El. B. to sub. orbit. Generally yields to a few electric applications.

260. Swelling soft-Without pain (anasarea), with weakness, thirst, diarrhoea, scantiness of urine.

Baths of A2. S. a b. s., and according to the case, F. a b. s. or C. a b. s. Baths of C5 or A2. El. R. "—" El. J. to occ., symp. plex. sol., also baths of El. B.

Treat, in the same manner, general swelling of the body.

Swelling of the hypochondres; F II a b. s. and onct. of F2, and baths of C5. El. R. "—" El. J. to symp., plex. sol., occ., onct. to the hypoc. of C5, comp. of El. B.

261. Syncope-See *Fainting Fits.*

262. Syphilis-Ven. internally and externally: C5, C4, A2 Ver. S. a b. s., repeated baths of C5. are very efficacious, and of S. A2. El. B. El. R Ven. and S5, comp. onct. of Ven. S5, 20 gr. C5, onct. to the hypoc. of F2 or C5, El. R. "—" El. J. to occ., symp., plex. sol. Injections and clysters, according to the case, of anticanceroso.

The distinctions made between primary and secondary syphilis have for us no absolute value. Syphilis is only one; the degrees of gravity, the difl'erent forms that it affects, the complication of symptoms, etc., all depend upon the dispositions of the organism which has absorbed the syphilitic virus. This is proved by the fact that one remedy is specific and chief in curing the alterations caused by syphilis. The other remedies, above indicated, act to support the antivenereo, a medicine which is fit to regenerate the human race. The cures, here, besides those reported by doctors Pascucci and Regard are really innumerable.

The following syphilitic complaints can, be attacked and radically destroyed by the medicines above indicated, namely.

The eruptions on the skin, nodes, (comp. of Ven.) old syphilis, weakness from venereal excess, bubo, falling away, wasting condylomata (syphilitic warts) deep wounds, inflammation of the inquinal glands, fetid ulcers.

Wounds with leathery edges, ulcers and ulcerations of the prepuce, hard ulcers with sharp edges, inflammation of the glands, pains in the bones, complicated inflammation of ganglion following on fatigue.

The chancre, hard or soft, blenorrhagia, primary syphilis, gonorrhea, drop discharges from the urethra, or vagina, stricture of the urethra, blenorrhoea, chronic inflammation of the urethra or vagina, syphilitic orchitis, adenitis, peeling of the epidermis, and daily fever, prepuce swollen, forced back with venereal warts on the glands, phagedenic chancres 0f the glands, the canal of the urethra raw, syphilitic abscesses of the skull, etc. It must be borne in mind that the remedy is to be attenuated in proportion to the gravity of the disease, and, also, that the anticancerous are necessary, in serious cases, to support the action of the antivenereal.

T

263. Teeth-Affections of the teeth in general. S. C. A. Onct. of C5. to the part affected by the pain. Gargles which may be alternated with the electricities red or white, angioitic or red.

a. *Receding of the gums*; wash the mouth with water in which is dissolved some C5. or 20 gr. of C5. Baths and onct of C5. Baths and onct. (to the jaw) of S. El. B. or El. A. in the mouth A. S.

b. *Toothache*. El. R to the external point of the pain; if of no effect, El. J. and onct. of C5. Baths of C5. S. Compr. El. B.

c. *Toothache, with swelling of the face*, see *b*.

d. *Difficult dentition*: to the nurse, S. or 10 gr. of A. Onct. of C5. to the infant's jaws, El. R. "—-" El. J. to massiter.

e. *Dental fistula*: as 263; also wash the mouth with 50 gr. of C5. dissolved in a glass of water. Onct. and compr. of F2. to the hypoc.

f. *Toothache* caused by cold; El. R. "—" El. J. ; compr. of El. B.

Diseases of the teeth cured by these means are innumerable.

264. Tenia-See *Worms*.

265. Testicles-Simple inflammation of the Testicles. Baths, onct , compr. of C5. CII. a b. s. 10 gr. of C5. Baths, onct., compr. of S. Compr. of El. B. El. R. "—" El. J. to the sacral nerves, pubis, perineum. A II. Onct., baths A2.

Veneral orchitis. Ven n. Compr. of Ven. onct., compr., baths of C5. of S. El. B. onct. of A2. C II a b. s. Compr. of C.

266. Tetanus, complete or partial-Compare Lockjaw. Partial tetanus has been relieved by El. J. to the occiput only; complete. by the same applied to the occ., symp., plex. sol. and all the affected nerves.

267. Throat-Laryngitis, inflammation of the larynx. S II. P II. C2. II alternated; gargles of El. B. C5. S. Baths of C5. S. A2. El. B. "—" El. J. to occ., symp., onct. of C5. to the hypoglosses A2 II.

a. *Rheumatic laryngitis*, as 267, also compr. C5. S5. and El. A.

b. *Angina pectoris.* Onct. to whole of the chest of C5. gargle El. R., with oppressed breathing-See *angina pectoris*; also compr. of A. to the heart, to sides of seventh vertebra (at the base of the neck, at the level of the shoulders; see diagram) and pit of the stomach. El. A. in same manner.

c. *Simple sore throat.* F II. a b. s. afterwards S. a b. s. gargle El. R. and El. B.

d. *Diphtheria.* C. a b. s. gargle of C. S. El. R. El. B. and El A.

e. *Affections of the windpipe*; as 267.

f. *Difficulty in swallowing*; as 267. El. R. "—" El. J. to great hypoglossids.

g. *Cancerous Tonsils*; as 267 frequent and abundant gargles.

h. *Clergyman's sore Throat.* S. "—" A II. gargle of El. B. or R. El. R. "—" El. J. to the hypoglos. See 267.

A weakened voice may be restored by El. R. to symp.

i. *Tumour of the pharynx*: see 267. Abundant gargles and onct. of C5. to the throat.

268. Tic douloureux, Neuralgia, Face ache-Onct. to part affected of C5. S. A. or El. R. "'—" El. J. compr. El. B. or El. A. or C. S. C4. A. A2. internally. Baths of C5. S. and A2.

269. Tongue (Cracks and inflammation of)-S II. C5. S5. a b. s. gargles of same remedies, or with El. B., or R. El. R. "—" El. J. to the hypogl. occ., or else baths, onct. (to hypogl.) of C5. and S. gargles of A2.

270. Tonsilities-Swelling, redness, and hardness of the tonsils. S. A. gargles with these remedies, (20 gr. to a glass of water.) Gargles of El. R. El. B. or El. A. Baths of C5 comp. of C5 to the external parts, chronic, the same treatment.

271. Tumors, Insensibility is a cancerous characteristic; in this case treat as cancer.

a. *Flashy, soft, moist, reddish vegetations*, (warts, condylomata, wens, etc., employ S. C5 A.

b. *Tumors of the breast, bones, knee*; see *Breast, nodes, knee.*

c. *Hydrocele*, Tumor of the scrotum from serious accumulation. C. A. A2. See *Cancer*.

d. *Varicocele*, tumor of the scrotum produced by dilation of the veins, A. A2. onct. of A2. onct., compr., baths of C5, baths of A2, compr. of A2. El. A. S. internally with onct. of same.

e. *Tumor of the cornea*: Staphyloma. S. C5. A. onct. of C5 compr., baths of the same, Baths of S., onct. compr. of S. over the closed eye. Onct. of A2. El. B. to the closed eye. El. R. "—" El. J. to occ., symp., super and sub. orbital. Onct to the hypoc. of F2 and C5.

Tubercular tumor of the belly: C. Baths, comp., onct. the belly of C5 20 gr. C5. Baths of S. A2 and S5, comp. of El. B. to the belly, El. R. "—" El. J to symp., plex. sol. and loins.

f. *Internal fibrous tumor*, giving the appearance of advanced pregnancy, but with decided hectic symptoms. C. and onct, to the hypoc. of F2. The rest as f.

g. *Cure of a scrofulous tumor of the thigh bone*, which was decayed in three parts, disease of nine years standing.

Cure of a tumor accompanied by serious disorganization of the ankle of the foot, (consequent on fracture,) and which it was proposed to amputate.

U

272. Ulcerations-see *cancer, scirrhus, skin.*

273. Ulcers, phagedanic, venereal or of syphilitic taint. See *Syphilis.*

a. *Scorbutic ulcers.* S. C. A2 C5 C4. Gargles with all these remedies. Baths of C5. S. A2 S5. Gargles of El. B. El. R. "—" El. J. to symp., occ. plex., sol. gargle of El. R. or El. A.

b. *Varicose ulcers.* See *varicose veins*, Onct., comp. A2. The same internally with baths of A2. Onct to the hypoc. of F2 or C5. Baths, onct. and comp. of C5.

274. Urethra-Congenital stricture. S. comp, onct. baths of S. baths onct., comp. to the urethra of C5 S5.

Comp. El. B. Injections of S. or C5 El. B. "—" El. J. to sacred nerves, pubis and perineum, Baths of El. B , or El. R.

Stricture of the urethra from external causes: as above-Cure of a man aged 53 years, and another of 39 years, afflicted with congenital stricture of this class.

275. Urine-See also *Bladder.*

a. *Albuminuria*, (urine charged with albumen, Bright's disease). C. C5. S. S5. a b. s. Baths of C5. S. A2. S5. El. B., or El. R. El. R. "—" El. J. to occ., symp., sacred nerves, and along the spine.

b. *Dysuria*; dilficulty in passing water. S2. A2 II. a b. s. 20 gr. C5. and as above.

c. *Diabetes.* (Urine charged with sugar.) See the word; select also the medicines a. and b. above, also onct. to the hypoc. of F2. and C5.

d. *Hoematuria*. (bloody urine.) A2 II. A II. S. II. a b. s. compr. onct., (to sacred nerves) baths of A2. comp. over the region of the heart with A. onct. to the hypoc. of F2. Baths of El. A. or El. B. El. R. "—" El. J. to occ., symp. plex. sol. and sacred nerves.

e. *Spermatorrhoea*, as a. and b., also see the word.

f. *Incontinence of urine*; see the word.

g. *Loss of urine*. S. a b. s. El. R. to the sacred nerves. El. R. "—" El. J. to same, or El. A. see *b*.

h. *Scalding urine*. See *a*. When there is, alternately, loss and difficulty of passing, follow the remedies indicated under letter *a*. The same for dysuria after the extraction of the foetus.

276. **Urine**, *Incontinence of*-S. 20 gr. of C5. A2. Baths of C5. S. A2. El. R. "—" El. J. to sacred nerves, to symp. Compr. of C5 to pubis, also of S. A2. El. B.

a. *The same* when produced by paralysis of the prostrate gland.

b. *In children*. Verm. El. B. to sacred nerves, to pubis. Compr. to pubis of A2. El. R. "—" El. J. to sacred nerves.

c. *Paralysis of the bladder*. Also 276, also injections of El. B. or A. onct. of C5. to pubis and perineum.

277. **Urine**, retention of-See *Bladder*.

278. **Uterus**-See *Womb*.

V

279. **Vaccination** maladies consequent on inoculation of the vaccine-S. and the remedies *275 a*.

280. **Vaginitis**-Inflammation of the nervous surface of the vagina, acute or chronic, and all its varieties (erythemathous papular, vessicular or eczematous.) C. II. C5. II. a b. s. Baths of C5. and compr. to pubis, perineum, and sacred nerves. Baths of S. and S5.

281. Varicose veins-Wounds, varicose ulcers, complicated with rheumatism, etc. treat by angioitics and by remedies *275 a.* add, also, baths and onct. G5.

a. *Old indurated varicose veins* of the knee, or abdomen, as *above*, also baths of C5. A2. onct. of C5. The cure is certain.

282. Vericocele-See *Tumors* and *Varicose veins.*

283. Vegetations, fleshy-See *Tumors*; treated under all forms by anticancerous, and antiangioitics.

284. Veins, affections of-Phlebitis, Phlegmasia, (Inflammation of) etc. See *Blood.*

285. Vertigo, from excess of blood-Employ the angioitics mentioned *275* letter *d.* Vertigo after miscarriage, C II. a b. 5. if proceeding from the spleen F II. a b. s. Onct. or compr. to the hypoc. of F2. C5.

286. Viper (bite of)-I have not yet treated such a case, but I think that the anti-scrofoloso expels the virus, from the reason of its action on other poisons.

287. Voice (loss of)-El. R. to occ., symp., plex. sol. especially to pit of stomach. Also El. A., or else El. R. "—" El. J. to the hypogl. and pit of the stomach. Gargles of El. B. S. A2. internally, baths of C5. A2. See also *Throat*, letter *h.*

288. Vomiting-S II a b. s. 10 gr. S. The same remedies also apply to the vomiting of pregnancy.

a. *Hoematemesis*, vomiting of blood, proceeding from the mucous membrane of the stomach, more or less, dark red in colour, A II. A2 II. a b. s. See also *Urine* letter *d. Hoematuria.*

b. *Hoemoptysis*; spitting of blood; a symptom, always connected with serious lesions of the chest, and frequently indicative of tubercular diathesis. It requires antiangioitics, pectorals (if there is cough) 7 and the medicines indicated, article *Lungs.*

c. *Meloena*; see the word; the cause, above all, must be studied, as it may be either a symptom of enterorrhage (exhalation of blood to the surface of the mucous membrane) or a specific disease, characterized by intense colics, paleness of the face, fainting, etc. The remedies must be selected conformably, employing small doses: See *Rectum*, loss of blood from.

d. *Continual vomiting* lasting 15 months, cured. In general, onct. to the hypoc. of F2. El. R. to bottom of stomach S II. a b. s. 10 gr. S. Baths of C5. S. comp. of El. B. to bottom of stomach El. R. "—" El. J. to plex. sol.. symp. and pit of stomach.

e. *Periodical vomiting*. F. II. a b. s. onct. to the hypoc. of F2. or C5. See *288*.

f. *Vomituration*. See *stomach*.

Cure of Vomiting in every form. Vomiting by the nose; daily, with diarrhoea, etc. In general, the remedies indicated *2-8* and letter *d*.

W

289. Warts-See *Tumours*.

290. Weakness-See *Debility*.

291. Whitlow-At the onset, try the abortive treatment by comp.El. B. or El. R. or baths, onct., comp of C5 after the commencement; if not arrested, treat with S II. C II. a b. s. comp. of S. or sometimes A2.

292. Whites see *womb* and *abdomen* letter *0*.

293. Womb (Pains in)-generally cease with first spoonful of C. or C II. Baths of C5. onct., comp. of same to the pubis. Baths of S. or A2 El. R. "—" El. J. to the sacred nerves and symp. comp. of El. B. to the sacred nerves. S. II.

a. *Metritis (puerperal)*-inflammation following after confinement. S. II a b. s. C. II a b. s. C5 II a b. s. or 10 gr. C5. Baths, onct., comp. to pubis of C5. El. R. "—" El. J. to sacred nerves, or baths of S5. or A2., El B. to pubis and sacred nerves.

b. *Ovaritis.* Inflammation of the ovaries. See *a*, also, onct, of C2 to the parts, and El. R. "—" El. J. to symp., plex. sol. and sides of the spine. If there is congestion S. III. a b. s.

c. *Ovaries* and all their diseases, C II a b. s. and the electricities as b.

d. *Polypus of the womb* (compare cancer) C II "—" A2 II. Baths, onct. (to pubis) comp. of C5 or A2. 20 gr. of C5 El R. "—" El. J. to sacred nerves. Comp. to pubis of El. B. Injections of C. C5. C4 A2 S5 S2. Baths of S., and in case of hoemorrhage baths of A2, comp. to heart of A.

e. *Falling of the Womb*; see *d*. also compr. of El. B.

f. *Spasms of the Womb*; see *293*.

g. *Retraction af the ligaments of the Womb*; see *d*.

h. *Chronic congestion of the Womb*; see *293*. and frequent injections as *d*.

i. *Granulations of the Womb*; see *d*.

j. *Nervous affections of the Womb*; see *Hysteria*, employ the 3rd dilution a b. s.

k. *Uterine melancholy*; see *j*.

l. *Uterine headaches*; see *j*. with light comp. of El. R. or B. to super orbitals.

m. *Hoemorrhage of the Womb*; see *Menses*.

n. *Change of life*; see *Menses* also S II. a b. s.

o. *Periodical colic of the Womb* F II a b. s.

p. *Disorders caused by painful labours*; see *d*.

q. *convulsions of the Womb* C III a b. s. the rest as letter *d*.

294. Worms-Ascarides, (thread worms) lombricoides (stomach worms) tenia, tape worm, tricocephale, etc. employ the vermifuges at the 1st or 2nd dilution according to the case.

a. *Disorder caused by worms*: Diarrhoea, vomiting, convulsions, etc. The vermifuges, and onct. and compr of F2, C5 to the hypoc.

b. *Tape worms*. Give, at first, a decoction of senna; the day after, commence by employing the vermifuges.

Sometimes, the expulsion of the worms shows them entire or in pieces, at others; these are not visible, although the state of health proves the cure. Ver 1, Ver 2 II. C5.

295. Wounds (To arrest the bleeding of)-comp. of El. A.

Afterwards, to complete the cure, S. C. A., comp. El. B., El. R. or El. A. Baths of C5, comp. of the same or baths and onct. of S. Baths, onct. and compr. of A2. onct. to the hypoc of F2.

296. Wounds gangrenous-C. A2, compr. of these remedies, baths, onct., compr. of C5, S. A2. compr. El. B , El. V., El. A. Baths, onct., compr. of S. El. R. "—" El. J. to corresponding nerves.

a. *Wounds resulting from burns*. As 296. Also large comp. of A. A2. C. C5. 04 , and especially S.

S. and S2. hasten the cicatrising. If there is pain, El. B. El. R. "—" El. J. to corresponding nerves.

b. *Large burns on the hip and knee*, patient given up after 6 months of useless treatment. Cured by C. alone given internally and externally.

c. *Wounds and swelling over the entire body*. (Cold humours) cured by C. II. a b. s. and strong comp. of C.

d. *Enormous scrofulous wounds*, cured by S. alone, internally and externally, and alternate comp. of El. B. El. A. El. R.

e. *Wound and swelling of the hand*. Cured by C. "—" S. internally and externally, and the electricities as *d*.

In conclusion, our aim, we have already stated, was not to report, here, either the number or the details of the diseases cured by the new Therapeutic ; we have only wished, in this catalogue (relying entirely on facts proved) to display its resources, so that it may be easy, for every one, to cmploy it ; again, may it be said that the catalogue is not an invariable formulary for all similar cases ; it is, only, a guide which should be consulted after becoming thoroughly imbued with the principles and nature of Electro homeopathy, such as we have shown them before.

We will finish by a general remark, namely, that in obstinate and rebellious maladies, an unexpected resource is frequently found in *anticanceroso* 5. Onct., made, with this remedy, to the hypoc., or with *febrifugo nuovo, or* 2, as also with *vermifugo* given in the dose of 10 globules, dry on the tongue.

Appendix

The facts, proclaimed by the new *medicine*, are certainly so marvelous, that, unless they have been witnessed, they form a subject of hesitation for some, and of disdain for others. This mistrust is only too well understood, at a time, when mystification and jugglery seem to dominate the world; but disdainful refusal ought, no longer, to be permitted to educated persons, who see new facts announced, every day, which, in a former age, would have appeared impossibilities.

The extraordinary discoveries, in physics, are no longer astonishing, yet; however, *physicians* have qualified, with the name of *hallucination*, the cures wrought by electro-homeopathy[1]. This would prove that medical science is very little advanced; some physicians do not, even, believe in the possibility of real discoveries in medicine.

When facts exist, the marvelous, which surrounds them, is not a reason of rejection; the only task of science is to endeavor to account for it. This is why we have introduced, here and there, theoritical considerations in this work; this is, also, why we add some further details, which, in the course of the essay, would have caused too much deviation from its general plan, which was, before all, to demonstrate the reality of the discovery, rather than to prove and explain it

1. See the pamphlet: La Scienza nuova del conte Cesare Mattei, e la Scienza vecchia del dottore C.; Casale-Monfer'rato. Paola Bertero 1878.

scientifically. Yet, we have not the pretention to present a theory of electro-homeopathy, which, in reality, does not require one; we expose, simply, a sketch which appears, to us, to connect known facts with the marvels that physicians have taken for clairvoyance.

Living beings draw from the exterior world the materials which serve to form their bodies, to develop and sustain the whole of their organs, the harmonious work of which characterizes life. Under the generic name of food, should be comprehended all matter capable of contributing to the structure of the organism and, thus, developing the phenomena which are adapted to the state of life.

These materials, once introduced into the digestive apparatus, undergo gradual transformations by the influence of the gastro-enteric fluids, until, after a certain time, a refined part of the alimentary mass is passed into the blood, whereas the insoluble residue accumulates in the lower folds of the intestinal canal, which finishes by getting rid of and throwing it out of the economy.

The refined part of the aliments, which is directed into the blood, carries, with it, the principles necessary to the construction of tissues, principles which, the blood, by its movement, is charged to distribute in all parts. But the fluid, drawn from the ailments, is not complete, and is not vivifying, as long as it is not united to oxygen; this is why, before passing into the course of the great circulation, the nourishing fluid charges itself with the atmospheric element in the cells of the lungs. Thence the blood, combined with oxygen, *becomes the plasm of tissues, and the potential agent of phenomena which, jointly, constitute the manifestation of the organic life of a being.*

The blood contains, so to say, all the life, in the same manner that the re-agents, placed in the cells of an electric battery, contain virtually the potential and all the effects of the electric current which springs forth when the circuit is completed.

Thus, the nutrition, the growth, the play of the apparatus of life; then, the dissolution, the return of the elements to the inorganic world, result from the combined work of the air and the alimentary matter; this is why every living being depends upon the soil and the atmosphere. Then, it must be added, that all these changes of absorbed materials are accomplished by means of a gradual and increasing oxydation, of which, the formation of the blood is the mean term, that if the tissues, the highest term, after which the more advanced degrees of oxydation tend to decomposition, that is to say, to bring back organized matter to the exterior world, under inorganic forms.

To sum up, the aliments form blood by oxidation, the blood by oxidation produces the tissues, these, by super-oxidation give rise, by the increasing instability of molecular groups, to the products of elimination which abandon the organism and, again, return to inanimate nature. The work of transformation, which changes the aliment into blood, commences at the entry of the digestive apparatus, at the contact of the salivary secretion, is continued in the stomach and intestinal canal, under the combined influence of the bile, the pancreatic, gastro-enteric juices, etc.; so that the passage of the food through the digestive organs, from the mouth to the opposite orifice, has for result the formation of the nutritive juice. The chyliferous vessels take it up, by capillary attraction, and endosmosis, in proportion as lt is produced, lead it into the thoracic canal, whence the flow of the circulation carries it on. Here oxygen intervenes which persues the series of transformations; where the work of the stomach finishes, commences that of the lungs and heart, and life purely vegetative, is the work or continual labor of the two fundamental organs.

To follow this physico-vital labor, it is necessary to indicate, first, the elements which the blood conveys, and which are incessantly furnished by the process of the gastro-enteric digestion. Blood is composed of water, albumen, sugar, fat, and mineral salts. Sugar, coming from the contact of the bile, pancreatic juice and the intestinal secretions, at first changes into fat; sacharine matters are only fat producing bodies, and it is, under this form, that they assume a place in nutrition. After this, the nutritive extract may be considered as a solution of albumen, fatty bodies and mineral salts in water.

Then the albumen, by a first degree of oxidation, changes into fibrin of blood, the oxidation ; continuing through the tissues, the fibrin is deposited and transformed into solid muscle. In fact fibrin can be produced by introducing oxygen into blood freshly extracted from the arteries; only fibrin thus obtained is amorphous, for form cannot exist, as far as we know, apart from the natural mould of the organism.

Albumen contains sulphur and phosphorous; by the partial combustion of the sulphur, the albumen is converted into *caseine*, the ulterior oxydation of which, through the course of the blood, gives rise to the formation of the sides of the sanguine vessels, to the connecting sub-cutaneous tissue, to the elastic ligaments, to the skin, and to the whole mass of matter distributed throughout the organism, which, on boiling, separates in the form of jelly. The skin, with its appartenancies, is only a species of crust of the oxidation of *caseine*, a crust which disappears and is renewed by the progress of successive oxidation.

As to the fatty bodies, it may be said that they assume a direct place in the lormation of tissues, which, without these, would be wanting in suppleness and elasticity. The different movements, which take place in all parts of the animal machine, would, everywhere, produce disorder, suffering and constraint, if the friction of the hard portions was not removed by interposition of the fatty and other similar bodies. Besides this, fat seems to be the principle which causes evolution: the white corpuscles of the blood, the first globules separated from the nutritive fluids which unite in clusters and granulations to form the utricular tissue, are composed of fat, enclosed in an excessively thin albuminous membrane.

Finally, the mineral elements of the blood rank, in the organism, as the means of forming the frame of the solid arts and the canvass of tissues; this can be prove by the incineration of the portions of the body, properly managed. Thus the entire organism results from the materials contained in the blood, the true starting point of all the tissues. Nothing except the form, is contained in the tissues which did not pre-exist in the blood; in its turn, the blood draws all its materials from the aliments, and there is nothing in the blood which is not found in the alimentary matters.

But the principles of the blood have not, all, the same destination in composition of the organism, on the contrary, every tissue appears to draw, only, that which is adapted to it, and to reject the rest; it is this species of selection which, properly, constitutes the curious phenomenon of assimilation, a phenomenon which has been explained, to a certain point, by the known laws of physics. In fact, the sanguine fluid, starting from the centre of the circulation, penetrates into the extremeties of the tissues, with a speed which goes on decreasing, in proportion to the diameter of the vessels, which branching out, more and more, seem to be eifaced and form, at their extremeties, extremely delicate and complicated network: the *capillary system.* It is, in these meshes, that the sanguine tide overflows, and its current, reduced to its slowest speed, is arrested ; the blood, then, passes from one point to another by a real *transudation.* Hence, it results that the materials, carried along, are not, everywhere, deposited in the same manner; on the contrary, there takes place a sorting out, a successive and fractional filtration ; the nutritive fluid, at each step, divests itself of principles which cannot pass through the pores of the tissue by which the transudation takes place. To these mechanical conditions of the system must now be added chemical attraction and affinity which intervene, without doubt, to arrest *similar* molecules, to place them and to regulate the arrangements which, jointly, form the different tissues. The laws of matter are, everywhere, the same; the asteroides of space, which turn from their course by the vicinity of the earth and fall, by attraction, towards the surface, and the corpuscles of the blood, which, during its course, fall into the meshes of the sorrounding tissues, obey the common law of attraction; and it is this law which explains the phenomenon, apparently so unlike, of the circulation of matter in space and in living atoms. But it will be remarked that the explanation,that we here give of *assimilation*, necessarily supposes an organic arrangement, or else a pre-established structural plan, without which, the organization of the elements, conveyed by the blood, cannot be understood. But there is the mystery of the creation, the point which escapes the known laws of matter; it is the principle called *Enormou* by Hippocrates, the *archea*, of Van Helmont, the *plastic force* of Cudwort, the *anemisma* of Stahal, the *vital principle* of Barthez: the principle, which probably will escape all the physiologists of the world, and all researches of philosophy, as well as the power of the microscope. But it need not be concluded from this, that: "this all powerful and inexplicable principle takes possession of the constituent parts of the body, destroys, in them, all tendency to conform to the laws of pressure, shock, the force of inertia, fermentation, and of putrefaction, etc., and submits them, only, to the laws of life, that is to say, maintains them in the state of sensibility and activity necessary to the preservation of the living being, in a dynamic almost spiritual state." (Hahneman) The vital principle cannot annihilate the properties and forces of matter; but this rinciple, being supposed present, and the structural plan being given, the arrangement of matter, in the organism, is a physico-chemical process which can be followed so far as to explain, by known laws, the organic transformation of matter.

We have said that the parts of the organism are formed and renewed by means of oxydation and it is by the same process, that the assimilated elements are consumed and, finally, ejected from the frame. Oxygen, is at the same time, both the creative and the destructive agent of the tissues composing the organism.

We can follow the formation of excremental or products of elimination which result from the progressive action of oxygen upon the elements of the blood.—The white corpuscules, six hours after their appearance in the blood, are found changed to the state of red globules; later on, they assume their place in the flesh ; finally at the end of three weeks, they are eliminated from the tissue, in the state of combustive products, become useless to the organism and incapable of sustaining its activities.

The first products of this muscular oxydation are announced by the appearance of creatine, creatinine, and acid inosic, nitrogenous compounds very much charged with oxygen. Their presence has even been discovered in the blood; by the process of oxydation these bodies pass into the state of uric acid and urea, which represent the highest point of the oxidation of muscle or fibrous tissue. The blood is divested of all these products in its passage through the loins; the urinary organs carry them out of the economy as fast as they are formed.

The rapidlty, also, with which this work is accomplished, for a long time prevented the discovery of its seat; but now that these products of reduction have been found normally in the blood and in living tissues, it may be said, in a general manner, that all surfaces of the organism, moistened by the blood, are the seat of the union of oxygen with the hystological principles; union, of which the result, is the formation of creatine, uric acid, and urea. They are not the only substances which represent the products of reduction, whose composition, it is understood, must vary, according to the nature of the tissue from which the elements all again. Thus the albuminoid and colloid bodies, scattered throughout the organism, give rise, in their union with oxygen, to the formation of *leucine*, a body which, in fact has been found in the salivary glands, in the pancreas, in the lungs, in the lymphatic glands, etc. either as a recrement, or as a recremento —excremental product.

The nitrogenous ternary bodies, compose of hydrogen, oxygen and carbon, such as sugar and fat, are also eliminated from the economy, by the labor of progressive oxidation, of which the last point is water and carbonic acid; whereas lactic acid, butiric acid, formic acid, oxalic acid, etc. represent the intermediate degrees of oxidation.

These products are, also, found in the economy, and can, also, be roduced in muscle, detached from the living body, by plunging it into oxygen; this, evidently, proves that their formation in the economy is entirely due to oxydation.

These new products leave the organism by different issues, namely : by the lungs, the loins, the entire surface of the skin; a part of the water and carbonic acid exhales, in the gaseous state, from the lungs and from the skin, by perspiration; the rest escapes by the urinary organs. The function of the skin is, here, analogous to that of the lungs; only, the latter absorbs more than it rejects. The intestinal canal assists, also, in the elimination of the products of reduction, as these products are found, in the state of mucous, mixed with the insoluble residue of the aliments.

The mineral principles, contained in the organism, of which we have stated, form the framework and the warping, are also re-exchanged, transformed and discharged, for the most part, by the urinary organs, in the state of carbonates, sulphates, phosphates, etc., and which are found abundantly in the urine. Finally, all parts of the body, which fall into disquamation: the hair, the nails, corns, etc., belong to the series of the products of slow and progressive combustion which works, without ceasing, in the midst of the organism and, by means of which, is affected the perpetual exchange of matter between the outer world and animated beings.

This matter, running through its circle, goes to form, first, atomical arrangements in the living tissues, arrangement of which the characteristic is instability and absence of crystalline forms ; it is, afterwards, resolved into different groups, during its return, grou s of which, the characteristic is a much greater stability of composition and the decided tendancy to the crystalline forms, proper to mineral matter.

We have only spoken of the transformation of the matter which traverses the living organism ; but the forces, themselves, which govern the working of the organic apparatus, result from these transformations, as will be seen. After the law, well known in this day, of the preservation of *live forces* in all the transformation of matter, the atoms, which fall from the blood and remain in the mass of the tissues, change their swiftness of removal, but they cannot lose the live force equivalent to their first movement. But it is this mechanical force, which, afterwards, appears as organico-vital force: each atom of blood which is fixed, deposits, in the midst of the organism, a quantity of vital energy, exactly equivalent to the lost motion, in the same manner as each atom of charcoal, that burns, develops a determined quantity of heat, and each particle of zinc, which is dissolved in an electric plate, throws, into the conductor, an equivalent quantity of electricity. Thus, the life force, existing in the atoms, at the moment they leave the blood, is found converted into the proper force of the organs to which the atoms are to be united, and of which, consequently, the working is the organico-vital equivalent of the atomic properties and energies. Whatever may be the difference between the two phenomena, it is sufficient to know that one is the result of the other to convince that an equivalence exists between them. But the working of the apparatus cannot take place without the action of the blood; then, the organico-vital phenomena, or else the working of each organ, represent the equivalent of live forces of the elements of blood which is, for this reason, called the *vivifying element*.

Equivalence does not, in general, entrain similitude; a weight, which falls, is far from being similar to heat; the solution of a metal, in a voltaic pile, is not similar to electricity; however, there is mathematical equivalence. In the same way, the transformation of the corpuscules of the blood have no resemblance with the vital phenomena which follow on. But, it is necessary that there should exist, also, a correlativeness of equivalence, as the organism cannot create nor annihilate anything.

But the phenomena of which the whole, jointly, constitutes the organic function, have, necessarily, a resemblance between themselves; and this function is only the continuous reproduction of a fixed order of phenomena; life, itself, in its entirety, is, only, a series of similar phenomena, succeeding each other without interruption. The reproduction of similar effects, of which one is the continuation of the other, on the one part; the re-exchange, on the other art, and the renewing of materials in the midst of which these effects are produced, lead us, forcibly, to suppose that there is a certain disposition, a certain arrangement of these materials necessary to the conditions of life. In other terms, it is necessary that the elements which leave the organism, and those which enter to replace them, be *similar*, that is to say, capable of developing the same energies, or, which is the same thing, of passing by the same change of forms, and of being reduced to the same products of secretion and excretion. The functions which, in their entirety, constitute organic life, can not be otherwise conceived.

Every phenomenon, which departs from the function natural to an organ, deranges life, and is a morbid phenomenon; its repetition and duration constitute a disease. Disease is not a defect, except for the living being; it does not affect matter which, whatever may be the order of transformations it follows, does, not the less, preserve its properties and forces. Disorder in the physiological functions or disease cannot be brought into the organs, but by materials or atoms which differ, in their mode of action, from those whose place they take in the tissues; the presence of the bodies which we may call *heteromorphous* and *heterodynamic*, has, for effect, the degeneration or transition, from the range of phenomena proper to life, to the range of phenomena of inorganic nature.

Every agent, capable of restoring its natural mode of action to the organism, is a *medicine*, and, after the preceding analysis, a medicine is the ponderable or imponderable matter, which, by its passage through the organs, re-establishes the natural functions when deranged, in whatsoever manner it may be. Then, in order that a matter acts thus, it is, above all, necessary that it reaches the point of the organism where the disorder has sprung forth : therefore *decided relations must exist between the therapeutic agent and the corruptive heteromorphous elements.*

The necessity of carrying the restorative principles to the very centre of the viciation or lesion is evident, as they must displace and expel those which have caused the mischief. On the other hand, known facts authorize us to state that a *certain similarity* is the condition necessary to enable two atoms to replace each other, and fill the same parts in the living tissues. We know, in fact, that the different materials, carried by the blood, are drawn, all of them, to homologous parts ; and the law, according to which these bodies are ranged and assimilated to one part more than another, depends, essentially, on the affinity and the atomatic configuration, in respect to texture of the network forming the organic woof irrigated and penetrated by the blood. In reality, it is the similarity and affinity which, in the process of nutrition, sort out the elements distributed in the blood. This is, why, the salts of soda, potass, phosphorous, etc., which the aliments discharge into the blood, mixed together, are soon separated, the soda going to the plasma, the potass to the globules, the prosphorous combines with the fatty bodies and afterward, with the nervous tissues. This is, then, a fact, a general law of the organism, that the different elements which traverse it, are separated from the liquid which carries them, directed towards and joined to their homologous centres, their to replace their similars. This, then, is the relation which ought to exist between the morbid principles and the therapeutic agent, proper to overthrow them ; this is, evidently, the reason of the *law of similars*.

Only, let the words be thoroughly understood, for it might be believed that a *similar remedy* could only add to the evil. Similarity is not *identity*, which is only a particular case of similarity. A similar, as regards our question, is matter capable of replacing, in the altered parts of the organism, the morbid principles found there, either in a latent state, or in one of morbid activity, and to form, by its substitution, new atomic groups of which it is possible, for the organism, to rid itself by its natural actions. We have seen that the organism renews and recasts its tissues, incessantly, by gradual transformation of the constituent elements; it is natural to believe that this work of renewal is deranged in the suffering or altered parts; the resistance to transformations, on which depends the organic vitality, is, necessarily greater in the heteromorphous elements, as these elements, no longer, revolve in the orbit of life and have not the same manners nor the same ways of dispersion.

This is why the restorative agent, although bringing similar elements of substitution, ought not to be indentical, as it would, then, only continue the same state of things. We, now, add that, after substitution, new atomic groups ought to be found, of which the organism can disengage itself, by means of its natural actions. Then, this is what ought to follow, as, on one hand, the labor, even of substitution, is the awakening of vital activity in the altered parts; on the other, the condition of a least fixity, of a least resistance to transformation, can always be realized, in the new combinations produced by the substitution of a similar.

This is, no more, than a question of dosology, and of attenuation of the matter, which is made to intervene in the place of the corruptive elements.

So, the similar medicine is placed between two classes of phenomena: disease and the normal state of organism; the result of its intervention is, at first, to lessen, then gradually destroy and, finally, expel the evil.

We shall not stay to develop the consequences of the principles set forth, of which every one can seize the theoretical importance, to make himself acquainted with the truths and the practice proclaimed by the newly discovered medicine, and specially with the fundamental axiom that: LIFE IS IN THE BLOOD, DISEASE IN ITS VITIATIONS, AND MEDICINE IN SIMILARS.

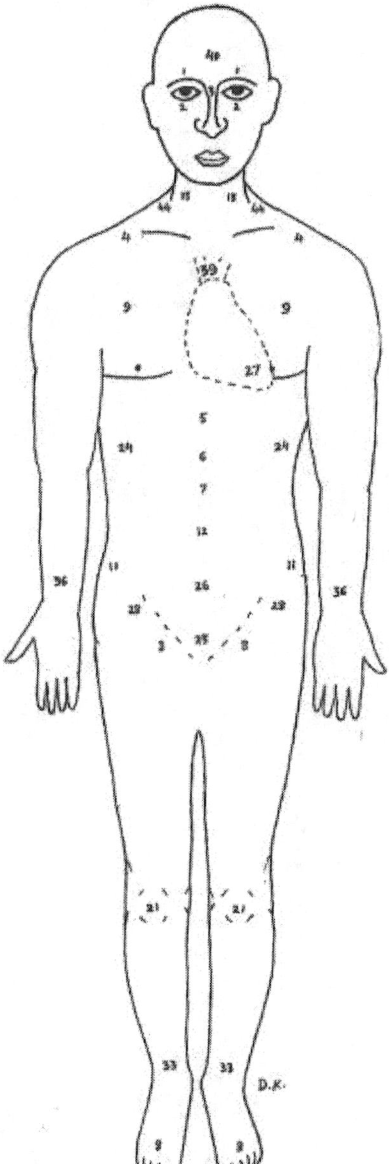

ANT VIEW *Points for Application*

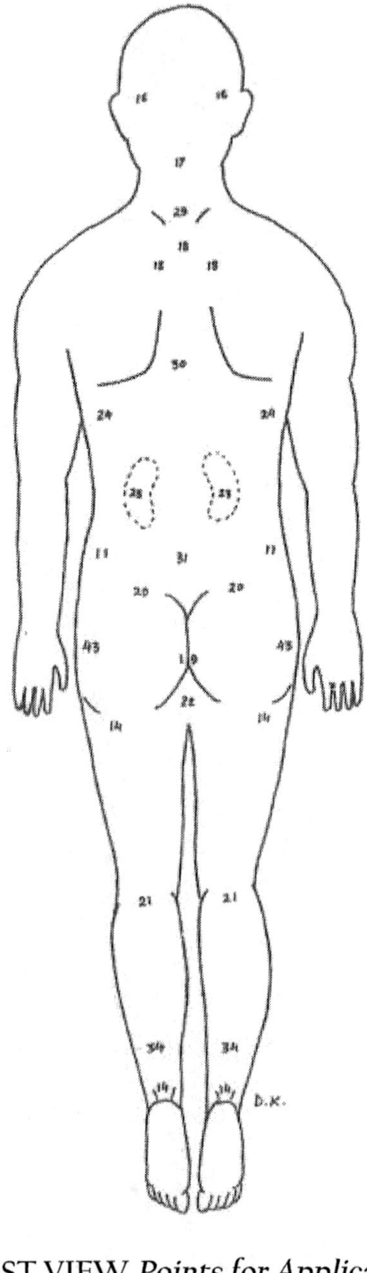

POST VIEW *Points for Application*

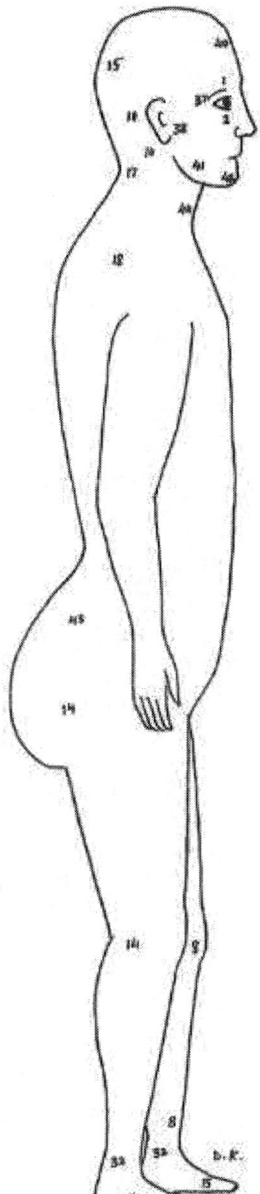

SIDE VIEW *Points for Application*